I0757378

Ashley Fitzgerald

STRESS HOLISTIC HEALING

Alternative Medicine for the Treatment of Stress

© 2024 by Ashley Fitzgerald
© 2024 by UNITEXTO

Published by UNITEXTO

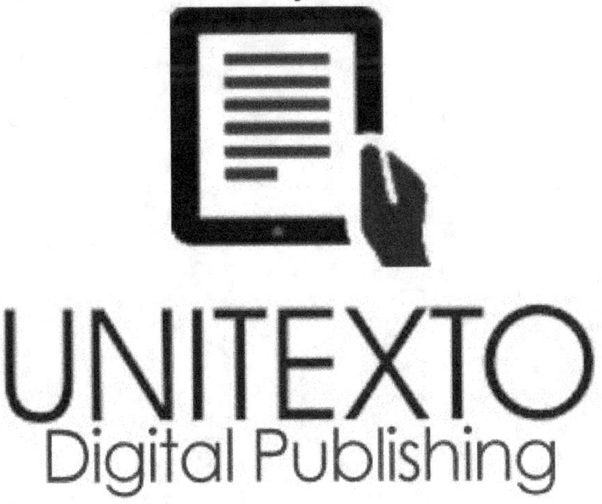

TABLE OF CONTENTS

Chapter 4: Meditation and Mindfulness Practices
- Introduction to meditation as a tool for stress relief and mental clarity
- Various meditation techniques for beginners and advanced practitioners
- Benefits of mindfulness in reducing stress, anxiety, and negative thought patterns
- Daily mindfulness exercises to incorporate into busy routines

Chapter 5: Somatic Therapy and Emotional Release
- Overview of somatic therapy and its role in releasing stored tension and trauma
- Techniques for tuning into bodily sensations to manage stress responses
- Exercises to connect mind and body, promoting a sense of calm and balance
- How somatic therapy complements other holistic practices

Chapter 6: Chakra Healing and Energy Balancing
- Introduction to chakras and their impact on physical and emotional well-being
- Identifying stress-related imbalances within each chakra
- Techniques for balancing chakras, such as visualization, sound healing, and essential oils
- The role of chakra healing in creating a holistic approach to stress relief

Chapter 7: Crystal Healing for Emotional and Physical Support
- Overview of crystal healing and the energies associated with different stones

- Selecting crystals to manage stress, improve sleep, and support mental clarity
- How to use crystals effectively: wearing, meditating, or placing them in specific spaces
- Creating a crystal toolkit for holistic stress management

Chapter 8: Feng Shui for a Calm and Peaceful Environment

- Introduction to Feng Shui principles and their impact on mental well-being
- Tips for arranging your space to promote relaxation and reduce stress
- Balancing the elements in your environment to foster harmony
- Simple adjustments in the home or workspace to improve energy flow and relieve stress

Chapter 9: The Power of Affirmations and Positive Thinking

- How affirmations influence the mind and reduce stress
- Developing personalized affirmations to support resilience and positivity
- Techniques to incorporate affirmations into daily life effectively
- The role of positive thinking in holistic stress management

Chapter 10: Oracles and Self-Reflection Tools

- Introduction to oracles (e.g., tarot, runes) as a method of self-reflection and stress relief
- How to use oracles for gaining insights, finding clarity, and managing stress
- The importance of intuition and inner guidance in holistic healing

- Practical exercises for using oracles in times of stress

Chapter 11: Creative Stress Relief: The Art of Tea and Adult Coloring
- Exploring the meditative aspects of traditional tea preparation and ceremony
- How the art of tea promotes relaxation, mindfulness, and calmness
- Benefits of adult coloring for stress relief and mental clarity
- Ideas for integrating creative outlets into a holistic healing practice

Chapter 12: Practical Wisdom for Lifelong Holistic Wellness
- Principles of practical wisdom for stress management and overall health
- Building a lifestyle centered on balance, simplicity, and inner peace
- Developing a long-term, personalized holistic health plan
- Final reflections on the benefits of a holistic approach to stress

Chapter 13. Weekly plan with activities for stress reduction

Chapter 14. Reference books for further research

Why this book?

In today's fast-paced world, stress has become a constant companion, affecting our physical, mental, and emotional health. Conventional medicine provides essential tools for treating the symptoms of stress, but many find these treatments alone insufficient for achieving long-term relief and inner peace.

This book, "Stress: Holistic Healing. Alternative Medicine for the Treatment of Stress", offers a fresh approach, focusing on complementary, holistic practices that treat the mind, body, and spirit as one interconnected system.

We created this book for those seeking a balanced, comprehensive guide to stress management, exploring various natural and alternative therapies that aim to harmonize the body's energy, restore emotional well-being, and foster resilience.

From understanding the roots of stress and its wide-ranging effects on health, to learning techniques for mindful living, each chapter introduces practices designed to reduce stress holistically, incorporating ancient healing traditions with modern insights.

Why this book? Because managing stress is more than just treating symptoms; it's about creating a lifestyle of well-being, exploring therapeutic methods that address the whole person, and empowering oneself to achieve lasting tranquility.

This journey emphasizes self-awareness, prevention, and the proactive nurturing of a balanced, peaceful life.

Whether you are new to holistic healing or looking to deepen your practice, this book offers an accessible path to rediscover peace in a demanding world.

Ashley Fitzgerald

About the Author

Ashley Fitzgerald: An Embodiment of Healing and Personal Triumph.

From a tender age, I, Ashley Fitzgerald, was acutely attuned to the nuances of health and personal well-being. These early inklings of self-awareness were not just passing contemplations but the seeds of a lifelong journey towards self-improvement and healing. As the chapters of life unfolded, I embraced my calling with fervor, transforming my youthful concerns into a robust career that spans two decades.

Today, I stand before you not merely as a practitioner but as a seasoned professional healer whose hands and heart have been instrumental in guiding countless individuals towards weight loss triumphs, enriched sexual health, and the surmounting of life's multifaceted challenges to reach the pinnacle of their health aspirations.

My professional and academic journey is a tapestry of diverse yet interconnected disciplines. With an insatiable thirst for knowledge, I delved deep into the realms of yoga and meditation, not just as practices but as academic pursuits, seeking to understand their profound effects on the human psyche and physiology.

This spiritual and intellectual quest further led me to the healing energies of Reiki, the organic wisdom in health foods, and the transformative potential of neuroscience and positive psychology. My foray into the science of health and exercise is not merely academic; it is a reflection of my intrinsic philosophy that the body and mind are inextricable partners in the dance of life.

My dedication to personal growth extends beyond my professional endeavors—it is a way of life. Each morning, as the world stirs awake, I find sanctuary in my daily rituals. My practice of yoga is more than a physical regimen; it is a journey towards achieving a state of zen-like tranquility, a testament to my belief in the power of simplicity and inner peace. Meditation accompanies yoga as my mental compass, guiding me through life's tumultuous waves with a steadfast calm.

What fuels my unyielding passion is an unwavering drive—an innate desire to not only absorb the myriad teachings that life has to offer but also to disseminate them. I am imbued with a relentless drive to unearth and share life strategies that spark a transformative flame within souls, urging them to reach for health, well-being, and the fruition of their deepest dreams.

It was this very desire that led me to the world of writing, to become a scribe of my experiences and insights. My pen is driven by a profound commitment to be a beacon of positivity, influencing the lives of others through words that resonate with truth and vitality.

As you turn the pages of my books, what you will find is a reflection of my heart's work. I invite you into my world, not just as a reader, but as a fellow traveler on this grand adventure of life.

Thank you for embarking on this journey with me, and it is my sincerest hope that you will find as much joy in reading my writings as I found in penning them down.

May the words you peruse inspire you to cultivate the health and happiness you so richly deserve.

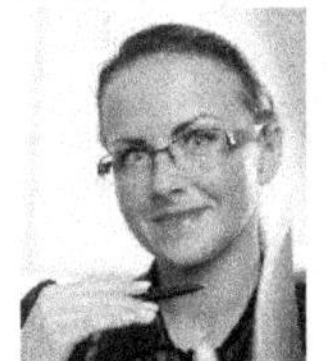

Ashley Fitzgerald

Chapter 1: Introduction to Holistic Healing

Holistic healing is a health approach that focuses on treating the whole person rather than simply addressing symptoms. Unlike traditional medicine, which often focuses on managing specific conditions or symptoms, holistic healing considers the interconnectedness of the body, mind, spirit, and emotions. This chapter provides an overview of holistic healing, explaining its principles and how it differs from traditional medical approaches. We'll also explore why holistic healing can be especially effective for managing stress and other health issues, while emphasizing the importance of integrating it with traditional healthcare.

Traditional vs. Holistic Approaches to Health

Traditional Medicine is grounded in scientific methods and primarily aims to diagnose and treat specific health issues. It is highly effective in treating acute conditions and has developed treatments for a wide range of diseases through medications, surgeries, and other medical interventions. For example, when someone suffers from asthma, traditional medicine provides inhalers and medications that can relieve symptoms almost immediately. However, traditional medicine often focuses on symptom relief and may not address underlying causes related to lifestyle, emotional well-being, or environmental factors.

Holistic Healing, by contrast, looks beyond symptoms and seeks to address the root causes of illness. In holistic health, the body, mind, spirit, and emotions are seen as interconnected parts of a person. If one area is unbalanced, it can affect overall health. Holistic approaches consider various lifestyle factors such as diet, stress, emotional health, and environment. As holistic healer and author Louise Hay famously said, "The body, like everything else in life, is a mirror of our inner thoughts and beliefs. Our bodies are always talking to us, if we will only take the time to listen."

Holistic healing utilizes a variety of natural and non-invasive techniques, such as herbal medicine, meditation, nutrition, acupuncture, and mind-body practices, which aim to create harmony and balance in the body. This approach also emphasizes prevention, encouraging individuals to adopt healthier lifestyles that promote long-term well-being. Holistic practitioners believe that by understanding and addressing the underlying causes of an issue, rather than merely treating symptoms, people can achieve sustainable health improvements.

Principles of Holistic Healing and Its Focus on Treating the Whole Person

Holistic healing operates on several core principles that differentiate it from traditional healthcare. Key principles include:

1. Interconnectedness:
   Holistic healing is based on the belief that each part of a person (body, mind, emotions, and spirit) is interconnected. Therefore, treating only one aspect of a person may not yield complete healing. For instance, an individual with chronic stress might experience not only mental exhaustion but also physical symptoms like

headaches and muscle tension, which are intricately connected.

2. Balance:
    Holistic health emphasizes the importance of maintaining balance in all areas of life. This principle is rooted in the idea that imbalance, whether emotional, physical, or spiritual, can lead to illness. By identifying and correcting imbalances through lifestyle adjustments and holistic practices, individuals can restore harmony and improve health.

3. Self-Healing:
    Holistic healing trusts in the body's natural ability to heal itself. Holistic practitioners believe that the body has innate wisdom and, when given the right conditions and support, it can often repair itself without aggressive interventions. Supporting the body through diet, rest, exercise, and emotional care can enhance its ability to heal.

4. Prevention:
    Prevention is central to holistic healing. Holistic practitioners encourage individuals to adopt practices that prevent illness rather than waiting to treat symptoms. This may involve managing stress, eating a nutritious diet, engaging in regular physical activity, and fostering positive emotional health.

5. Empowerment and Personal Responsibility:
    Holistic healing places a strong emphasis on the individual's role in their own health.

Practitioners often work to empower clients, helping them make informed choices about their lifestyle and health practices. This empowers individuals to take personal responsibility for their health rather than relying solely on external interventions.

According to Dr. Deepak Chopra, a prominent advocate of holistic medicine, "The mind and body are like parallel universes. Anything that happens in the mental universe must leave tracks in the physical one." This perspective underscores holistic healing's emphasis on viewing health as an intricate system, where each component—mental, physical, emotional, and spiritual—is equally significant and must be nurtured.

Why Holistic Healing Can Be Effective for Managing Stress and Related Health Issues

One of the primary benefits of holistic healing is its effectiveness in managing stress, which is both a common and pervasive issue. Research shows that chronic stress is linked to various health issues, including cardiovascular diseases, asthma, digestive problems, and weakened immune function. Unlike traditional approaches that may treat only the physical symptoms of stress-related illnesses, holistic healing addresses the root causes of stress by promoting relaxation, resilience, and balance.

Holistic healing often employs mind-body practices such as mindfulness, meditation, yoga, and breathwork, all of which are effective for reducing stress and promoting emotional well-being. Meditation, for example, has been shown in studies to reduce cortisol levels (the "stress hormone") and promote relaxation by activating the parasympathetic nervous system, which helps the body relax and recover. A study published in the Journal of Clinical Psychology found that regular meditation practice helped participants reduce perceived stress and increased their sense of calm and control over their lives (Kabat-Zinn, 1990).

Furthermore, holistic approaches often incorporate nutrition and herbal remedies that support physical resilience against stress. Adaptogenic herbs like ashwagandha, rhodiola, and holy basil, for instance, have been found to help the body adapt to stress by modulating the stress response system. Nutritional adjustments can also boost immune function and overall vitality, making individuals more resilient to stressors.

Holistic healing can also help individuals become more aware of their emotions and develop strategies for managing negative emotions that contribute to physical symptoms. Emotional well-being is often neglected in traditional medicine, but holistic practices recognize that emotions are stored in the body and can manifest as physical symptoms if left unresolved. Techniques like journaling, art therapy, and talking therapies can facilitate emotional release and help individuals understand and process their feelings in a healthy way.

The Complementary Role of Traditional Healthcare and the Importance of Consulting Medical Professionals

While holistic healing offers valuable benefits, it is essential to recognize that it is not a replacement for traditional healthcare. Instead, holistic practices can serve as complementary therapies that work alongside conventional medical treatments. In cases of chronic or serious conditions such as asthma, diabetes, or heart disease, traditional medicine's advanced diagnostic tools and treatments play an irreplaceable role in managing and treating these conditions.

A balanced approach to health often involves integrating traditional and holistic practices. For instance, someone with asthma might rely on inhalers prescribed by their doctor to manage acute symptoms while using holistic practices like breathwork, diet, and meditation to support overall lung health and reduce stress triggers. Dr. Andrew Weil, a pioneer in integrative medicine, emphasizes this point: "Integrative medicine neither rejects conventional medicine nor accepts alternative therapies uncritically. Instead, it considers both approaches and uses whichever treatments are safe and effective."

The importance of consulting medical professionals before pursuing holistic therapies cannot be overstated, especially when treating serious or chronic conditions. Certain holistic practices may interact with medications or exacerbate symptoms if not applied correctly. By consulting with healthcare providers, individuals can develop a balanced and personalized approach that incorporates the benefits of both traditional and holistic treatments. Practitioners trained in integrative medicine are especially well-equipped to help patients navigate these options safely.

Case Study:

Maria's Experience with Integrating Holistic Healing into Her Health Journey

Maria, a 52-year-old woman with chronic migraines, had been seeking ways to manage her symptoms beyond prescription medication. Although her medications provided temporary relief, her migraines were frequent and affected her quality of life. After consulting with an integrative health practitioner, Maria was introduced to holistic methods such as meditation, dietary adjustments, and acupuncture to help manage her migraines.

Maria began meditating daily, using guided visualization techniques to reduce stress and focus on releasing tension in her head and neck. She also made dietary changes by incorporating more anti-inflammatory foods like leafy greens, turmeric, and ginger, which are believed to help reduce migraine frequency.

Over several months, Maria found that her migraine frequency decreased significantly. Although she still used her prescribed medication for acute attacks, the holistic approaches provided additional, consistent relief. "Holistic healing changed the way I view my health," she reflected. "I'm no longer just treating symptoms; I'm understanding the deeper factors that contribute to my well-being."

Conclusion

Holistic healing offers a powerful and comprehensive approach to health by addressing the body, mind, spirit, and emotions as interconnected components. While traditional medicine excels at treating acute symptoms and life-threatening conditions, holistic healing focuses on creating a balanced lifestyle that supports long-term well-being. Through practices that promote relaxation, emotional health, and self-awareness, holistic healing is particularly effective for managing stress and its associated health issues.

However, it's crucial to approach holistic healing as a complement to, rather than a replacement for, traditional healthcare. By working together, holistic and traditional medicine can offer a more integrated, patient-centered approach to health, empowering individuals to actively participate in their healing journey while benefiting from the strengths of both worlds.

Chapter 2: Understanding Stress and Its Impact on Health

Stress is a pervasive aspect of modern life, and while a certain amount of stress can motivate and push us towards achievement, chronic stress has a profound impact on health. This chapter explores the physiological effects of stress, its influence on various bodily systems, and the importance of managing it to sustain long-term well-being.

Definition of Stress and Its Physiological Effects

Stress, as defined by the American Psychological Association (APA), is a "normal reaction to everyday pressures, but can become unhealthy when it upsets your day-to-day functioning." Hans Selye, a pioneering endocrinologist who studied stress, defined it as "the nonspecific response of the body to any demand made upon it." Selye's research found that stress triggers a sequence of physiological responses known as the General Adaptation Syndrome, which consists of three stages: alarm, resistance, and exhaustion. These stages illustrate how the body responds to stress over time, from an initial "fight or flight" reaction to a prolonged period of coping, and ultimately to a stage of burnout when resources are depleted.

In the alarm phase, the body reacts to a stressor by releasing cortisol and adrenaline. These hormones increase heart rate, blood pressure, and blood sugar levels, equipping the body to respond to perceived threats. While this response can be lifesaving in emergency situations, the persistent release of stress hormones can have detrimental effects, as highlighted in The End of Stress by Don Joseph Goewey (2014). Goewey explains that chronic stress keeps the body in a heightened state of alert, preventing it from returning to homeostasis and leading to what he calls "brain burnout."

How Chronic Stress Impacts Physical, Mental, and Emotional Health

Chronic stress goes beyond temporary discomfort; it reshapes the way our bodies and mind's function. This prolonged exposure can lead to numerous physical, mental, and emotional health issues.

Physical Health Impacts

The physiological effects of chronic stress are well-documented. Dr. Gabor Maté, a physician known for his work on mind-body unity, argues in When the Body Says No (2003) that stress suppresses the immune system, increases inflammation, and alters hormonal balances, making the body more susceptible to illnesses. This explains why people experiencing high levels of stress often report frequent colds, muscle pain, and even heart problems.

For example, a case study involving Sarah, a 45-year-old executive facing chronic work stress, showed that her consistent migraines, digestive problems, and muscle tension were directly correlated with her stress levels. Once Sarah began working with a therapist to manage her stress, her physical symptoms gradually diminished. This case emphasizes the role of mental well-being in physical health, illustrating the need for stress management to maintain overall wellness.

Mental and Emotional Health Impacts

Chronic stress also affects the brain, particularly in regions responsible for memory, emotion, and executive function. According to Dr. Robert Sapolsky, a neuroscientist who studies stress, prolonged exposure to stress hormones like cortisol can damage the hippocampus, which is crucial for memory and learning. Sapolsky, in his book Why Zebras Don't Get Ulcers (1994), explains that animals experience stress only momentarily in response to direct threats, whereas humans, due to our complex cognition, often experience stress continuously. This chronic state leads to cognitive impairments, anxiety, and even depression.

In a clinical study involving patients with generalized anxiety disorder, Dr. John Kabat-Zinn, a pioneer of mindfulness-based stress reduction (MBSR), found that incorporating MBSR significantly improved participants' mental health by reducing cortisol levels and enhancing emotional resilience. Kabat-Zinn's approach shows the promise of mindfulness and stress management for mental well-being.

Connection Between Stress and Illnesses

Stress not only affects mental health but can also manifest physically, leading to a variety of illnesses. Some of the most common stress-related issues include digestive problems, sleep disorders, hormonal imbalances, and autoimmune conditions.

Digestive Issues

The gut-brain axis, the biochemical signaling between the gastrointestinal tract and the central nervous system, is highly susceptible to stress. Studies published in the Journal of Clinical Gastroenterology show that stress can exacerbate digestive disorders such as irritable bowel syndrome (IBS) and acid reflux. A well-documented case involves Tom, a 30-year-old who was diagnosed with IBS shortly after starting a high-stress job. His symptoms included abdominal pain, bloating, and frequent digestive distress, all of which improved when he began a regimen of mindfulness practices and dietary adjustments under medical supervision.

Sleep Disorders

The interplay between stress and sleep is bidirectional: stress can lead to sleep disturbances, and lack of sleep can worsen stress. According to a study published in Sleep Medicine Reviews, chronic stress disrupts the normal sleep cycle by keeping the body in an alert state, leading to insomnia and poor sleep quality. This was observed in a case study involving Maria, a university student who reported frequent sleepless nights due to academic pressures. By incorporating relaxation techniques such as meditation and regular exercise, Maria saw a significant improvement in her sleep quality.

Hormonal Imbalance

Chronic stress disrupts the delicate balance of hormones, including cortisol, adrenaline, and sex hormones like estrogen and testosterone. Dr. Sara Gottfried, in her book The Hormone Cure (2014), argues that stress-induced hormonal imbalances can lead to weight gain, mood swings, and even reproductive health issues. For instance, Carla, a 35-year-old woman with chronic stress, experienced irregular menstrual cycles and mood fluctuations. When she implemented stress reduction strategies such as yoga and dietary changes, her symptoms gradually subsided, illustrating the impact of stress on hormonal health.

Autoimmune Disorders

Stress has been implicated in autoimmune disorders, where the immune system mistakenly attacks healthy tissues. In The Autoimmune Solution by Dr. Amy Myers (2015), it's argued that stress can trigger or worsen autoimmune responses due to its inflammatory effects. Research published in the Annals of the Rheumatic Diseases found that individuals with high stress levels were more likely to develop rheumatoid arthritis. Case studies of patients who reduced stress through meditation, lifestyle changes, and support groups reveal improvements in symptoms, emphasizing stress management's role in managing autoimmune conditions.

Recognizing Signs of Stress and the Importance of Managing It for Long-Term Well-being

Recognizing signs of stress early on is crucial for preventing long-term health problems. Common symptoms of chronic stress include headaches, muscle tension, digestive issues, fatigue, irritability, and sleep disturbances. According to the World Health Organization, "stress is the health epidemic of the 21st century." Despite its prevalence, many people normalize these symptoms, attributing them to aging or lifestyle without considering the role of stress.

Early Warning Signs

Dr. Andrew Weil, a leading figure in integrative medicine, suggests that early warning signs of stress may include subtle changes in mood, energy levels, or sleep patterns. In his book Spontaneous Happiness (2011), Weil emphasizes the importance of self-awareness and suggests practices such as mindfulness and deep breathing exercises to address stress in its early stages.

Case Study: Recognizing and Addressing Chronic Stress

Consider Jane, a 50-year-old teacher who initially attributed her fatigue, irritability, and occasional stomach pains to menopause. Over time, her symptoms worsened, affecting her ability to focus and enjoy life. After speaking with her doctor, Jane learned that stress was a significant contributing factor. Through a holistic approach that included counseling, diet modifications, and regular yoga, Jane was able to regain her energy and well-being. Jane's story underscores the importance of recognizing stress and actively managing it before it escalates into more severe health issues.

Long-Term Benefits of Stress Management

Managing stress is not merely about reducing symptoms but about cultivating a balanced and resilient approach to life. In The Relaxation and Stress Reduction Workbook (Davis, Eshelman, and McKay, 2008), practical techniques like progressive muscle relaxation, guided imagery, and self-compassion exercises are recommended for long-term stress relief. Dr. Herbert Benson, a pioneer in mind-body medicine, refers to this approach as the "relaxation response," a physiological state that counters the stress response and restores the body to equilibrium.

Practices like meditation, mindfulness, regular exercise, and a balanced diet contribute to building resilience against stress. This is supported by research published in Psychosomatic Medicine, which highlights that individuals who engage in regular stress management activities report improved mental health, reduced inflammation, and lower risk of chronic illnesses.

Quotations from Experts and Conclusion

Renowned psychotherapist Virginia Satir once said, "Life is not the way it's supposed to be. It's the way it is. The way you cope with it is what makes the difference." This quote encapsulates the essence of stress management: while we may not control all external circumstances, we can control how we respond to them.

Similarly, Carl Jung observed, "Even a happy life cannot be without a measure of darkness, and the word 'happy' would lose its meaning if it were not balanced by sadness." These perspectives emphasize that stress is an inevitable part of life, but managing it is essential for maintaining a balanced and fulfilling life.

By recognizing the signs of stress and addressing them proactively, individuals can significantly improve their physical, mental, and emotional well-being. While stress management may look different for each person, the underlying goal remains the same: to foster a balanced approach to life where health, happiness, and resilience are prioritized.

Chapter 3: Food Therapy for Stress Management

Food is a foundational element of holistic health, playing a crucial role in our physical, mental, and emotional well-being. In this chapter, we'll explore how food therapy can support stress management, examining the relationship between nutrition and stress, foods that promote relaxation and mental clarity, personalized nutrition plans, and strategies for identifying and managing food sensitivities that may worsen stress.

The Role of Nutrition in Holistic Health and Stress Reduction

Nutrition influences every aspect of our health, from energy levels and immunity to mood and cognitive function. The brain and body need certain nutrients to function optimally, and an imbalance in any one area can lead to stress or exacerbate existing stress symptoms. Dr. Mark Hyman, a leading expert in functional medicine, emphasizes in his book Food: What the Heck Should I Eat? (2018) that a balanced diet is essential for maintaining physical and mental health, as "food can either be the slowest form of poison or the most powerful form of medicine."

When we're stressed, the body releases cortisol, which can lead to increased cravings for sugary and high-fat foods. However, this "stress eating" often leads to energy spikes and crashes, worsening stress in the long term. By making mindful food choices that support energy balance, mood stabilization, and cognitive clarity, we can use nutrition to help manage stress more effectively.

In a case study involving Emma, a 30-year-old marketing professional dealing with chronic work stress, dietary adjustments were shown to significantly reduce her anxiety and mood swings. Emma replaced sugary snacks with complex carbohydrates, leafy greens, and foods rich in omega-3 fatty acids. Over the course of several months, she reported feeling more energetic and less prone to midday crashes, and her anxiety levels dropped considerably.

Foods That Promote Relaxation, Energy Balance, and Mental Clarity

Research has shown that certain foods have unique properties that promote relaxation, balance energy levels, and enhance mental clarity, making them excellent additions to a diet aimed at managing stress.

Foods Rich in Omega-3 Fatty Acids

Omega-3 fatty acids are essential for brain health and mood regulation. A study published in Brain, Behavior, and Immunity demonstrated that omega-3 fatty acids can reduce inflammation and lower cortisol levels, helping the body manage stress. Salmon, chia seeds, walnuts, and flaxseeds are excellent sources of omega-3s. Dr. Andrew Weil, a renowned integrative medicine specialist, recommends these foods for their anti-inflammatory effects and ability to support overall well-being.

Magnesium-Rich Foods

Magnesium is often called the "anti-stress mineral" because of its role in calming the nervous system. Studies published in the Journal of the American College of Nutrition have shown that magnesium can improve sleep quality, reduce anxiety, and relax muscles. Foods like leafy greens, almonds, and avocados are rich in magnesium. In a case involving Tom, a university student facing exam-related stress, incorporating magnesium-rich foods helped reduce his anxiety and improve his sleep quality, which positively impacted his overall performance.

Probiotic Foods

The gut-brain axis plays a significant role in stress management, with probiotics helping to maintain a healthy gut microbiome, which is linked to lower levels of anxiety and depression. Fermented foods such as yogurt, kefir, sauerkraut, and kimchi are rich in probiotics. According to a study in Psychiatry Research, participants who consumed probiotic-rich foods regularly experienced improved mood stability and reduced stress levels. Dr. David Perlmutter, in his book Brain Maker (2015), emphasizes that "gut health is brain health" and advocates for including probiotic foods to maintain mental resilience.

Complex Carbohydrates

Complex carbohydrates provide a steady source of energy, preventing the rapid blood sugar spikes and crashes associated with simple sugars. Foods like whole grains, oats, quinoa, and sweet potatoes support stable blood sugar levels, which in turn helps regulate mood. A study in Nutrition Research found that individuals who consumed complex carbohydrates regularly reported less anxiety and higher energy levels. This was particularly beneficial in the case of Carla, a busy entrepreneur who found that shifting to a whole-food, complex-carb diet made her feel more focused and less irritable throughout her workday.

Herbal Teas

Herbal teas such as chamomile, lavender, and passionflower have calming properties that can reduce anxiety and promote relaxation. A study published in Phytomedicine found that chamomile, in particular, has mild sedative effects, helping to reduce anxiety without causing drowsiness. Consuming a cup of chamomile tea before bed is a simple yet effective strategy for reducing stress and improving sleep quality.

Personalized Nutrition Plans to Support Resilience Against Stress

Personalized nutrition, or tailoring one's diet to individual needs and preferences, is key in holistic stress management. According to Dr. Lisa Mosconi, a neuroscientist and author of Brain Food (2018), "What you eat can affect how you feel, think, and perform every single day." Personalized nutrition takes into account unique factors such as genetics, lifestyle, and health conditions, allowing individuals to create dietary plans that suit their specific needs.

For example, someone with high anxiety may benefit from omega-3-rich foods, magnesium, and probiotics, while someone dealing with fatigue may prioritize complex carbohydrates and iron-rich foods. Personalized nutrition plans may also incorporate supplements, such as B vitamins, which are known to support mood and energy, or adaptogenic herbs like ashwagandha, which can help the body adapt to stress.

In the case of Daniel, a 45-year-old executive experiencing burnout, his nutritionist designed a plan high in lean protein, leafy greens, and antioxidant-rich berries. After three months, Daniel reported feeling more balanced, with fewer energy crashes, and improved resilience against work-related stress.

Steps for Creating a Personalized Nutrition Plan

1. Identify Goals: Establish clear goals based on stress management needs (e.g., better sleep, energy stability, improved mood).
2. Choose Key Nutrients: Select foods rich in nutrients that align with these goals, such as magnesium for relaxation, omega-3s for mental clarity, and complex carbs for steady energy.
3. Meal Planning: Plan balanced meals that incorporate these foods, allowing for flexibility to accommodate cravings and dietary needs.
4. Monitor and Adjust: Keep track of progress and make adjustments based on how different foods impact stress levels and overall well-being.

Tips for Identifying and Managing Food Sensitivities or Intolerances That May Exacerbate Stress

Food sensitivities can exacerbate stress by triggering inflammation, digestive discomfort, and mood changes.

For those with food sensitivities, stress management can become more challenging, as certain foods may worsen anxiety or irritability. Identifying and managing these sensitivities is essential for a holistic approach to stress reduction.

Common Food Sensitivities Related to Stress

Common culprits include gluten, dairy, and processed sugars, which can lead to bloating, fatigue, or mood swings in sensitive individuals. In a case study involving Linda, a 38-year-old experiencing chronic fatigue and anxiety, removing gluten and dairy from her diet under a dietitian's guidance led to a remarkable reduction in her symptoms. Her stress levels dropped as she no longer experienced the discomfort and fatigue previously associated with her meals.

Steps for Identifying Food Sensitivities

1. Elimination Diet:
   Temporarily remove common trigger foods (e.g., gluten, dairy, soy) and gradually reintroduce them to identify reactions.
2. Keep a Food Journal:
   Record meals and note any symptoms to track patterns and correlations between specific foods and stress-related symptoms.
3. Consult a Professional:
   Work with a nutritionist or allergist to confirm sensitivities through tests or structured diet plans.

Quotes and Perspectives from Experts

Famous therapists and nutrition experts alike have highlighted the importance of nutrition in managing stress. Dr. Elson Haas, author of Staying Healthy with Nutrition (2006), states that "nutrition is the foundation of healing" and "food is one of the most powerful tools we have to take control of our health." Haas emphasizes the holistic perspective, where food supports not only physical but also mental and emotional well-being.

Similarly, clinical psychologist Dr. Leslie Korn, author of Nutrition Essentials for Mental Health (2016), points out that "the right foods can heal the mind," and advocates for "nutritional strategies tailored to support mental clarity, focus, and emotional stability." Dr. Korn's work underscores the link between mental health and nutrition, emphasizing that food can act as a preventive measure against stress-induced mental health issues.

Conclusion

Food therapy is a powerful, natural way to manage stress holistically. By understanding how nutrition influences the body and mind, we can make food choices that promote relaxation, energy balance, and mental clarity. From magnesium-rich foods that calm the nervous system to probiotic-rich options that support gut health, food therapy offers diverse strategies for stress management.

A personalized nutrition plan, designed around individual goals and sensitivities, can further enhance resilience against stress. By paying attention to the foods we eat and their effects on our well-being, we can create a sustainable and balanced approach to managing stress.

This approach aligns with the holistic philosophy that health is a multifaceted state of well-being encompassing body, mind, and spirit. When we nourish ourselves mindfully, food becomes more than fuel—it becomes a vital tool for achieving balance and flourishing in the face of life's challenges.

Chapter 4: Meditation and Mindfulness Practices

Meditation and mindfulness practices have been used for centuries as tools for achieving mental clarity, emotional balance, and inner peace. Today, these practices are widely recognized for their role in managing stress, reducing anxiety, and cultivating a positive outlook on life. In this chapter, we'll delve into meditation as a transformative tool for stress relief, explore various meditation techniques suited to both beginners and advanced practitioners, discuss the science-backed benefits of mindfulness, and offer daily mindfulness exercises to incorporate into busy routines.

Introduction to Meditation as a Tool for Stress Relief and Mental Clarity

Meditation is an ancient practice that trains the mind to focus and calm itself, often by directing attention to a specific object, thought, or sensation. According to Jon Kabat-Zinn, a pioneer in mindfulness-based stress reduction (MBSR), meditation allows us to "find a sense of inner peace and balance amidst the chaos." Kabat-Zinn developed MBSR to help patients manage chronic pain and stress, demonstrating that meditation could be integrated into Western healthcare with significant success.

Physiologically, meditation reduces stress by activating the body's parasympathetic nervous system, also known as the "rest and digest" response. When we meditate, cortisol levels decrease, heart rate slows, and the mind enters a relaxed state. This counters the "fight or flight" response, which is the body's automatic reaction to stress. Dr. Herbert Benson, a Harvard physician, refers to this as the "relaxation response," a natural antidote to stress that meditation helps trigger.

Consider the case of Amy, a 35-year-old teacher overwhelmed by work and personal obligations. Amy struggled with anxiety, sleeplessness, and frequent headaches until she began a simple, ten-minute meditation practice each day. Over time, Amy noticed a profound change in her mental clarity, energy, and resilience against stress. Her story illustrates how meditation can serve as a powerful tool for fostering well-being in the face of life's demands.

Various Meditation Techniques for Beginners and Advanced Practitioners

There are many types of meditation, each with unique characteristics and benefits. Below are some techniques suited to different levels of experience.

1. Mindfulness Meditation

Mindfulness meditation, one of the most accessible forms, involves focusing on the present moment, usually by paying attention to the breath. This technique encourages a nonjudgmental awareness of thoughts and sensations, which helps reduce stress and anxiety.

A study published in Clinical Psychology Review shows that mindfulness meditation can reduce symptoms of anxiety and depression by promoting a sense of self-awareness. Mindfulness meditation is ideal for beginners due to its simplicity and adaptability. Practitioners can sit quietly, close their eyes, and focus on their breath, bringing their attention back whenever it wanders.

2. Guided Meditation

Guided meditation, as its name suggests, involves listening to a teacher or recording that provides instructions. This technique is beneficial for beginners who need help focusing or are uncomfortable with silence. Guided meditations often incorporate visualizations or positive affirmations to enhance relaxation and emotional well-being.

A case study involving Sarah, a nurse dealing with job-related stress, demonstrated the effectiveness of guided meditation. By listening to guided sessions during her lunch breaks, Sarah noticed a significant reduction in her stress levels and an increase in her emotional resilience.

3. Transcendental Meditation (TM)

Transcendental Meditation is a structured form of meditation where practitioners repeat a specific mantra to quiet the mind. Developed by Maharishi Mahesh Yogi, TM involves two 20-minute sessions per day and is known for its calming effects on the nervous system.

Research published in Psychosomatic Medicine found that TM lowers blood pressure and reduces stress more effectively than some other forms of meditation. TM is ideal for those who are committed to a more intensive daily practice and can benefit from a mantra-based approach.

4. Loving-Kindness Meditation (Metta)

Loving-kindness meditation, or Metta, is a practice focused on cultivating feelings of compassion and kindness, both towards oneself and others. By repeating phrases such as "May I be happy, may I be healthy, may I be at peace," practitioners learn to foster positive emotions and empathy.

Dr. Kristin Neff, a psychologist known for her work on self-compassion, found that loving-kindness meditation helps reduce self-criticism, anxiety, and negative thought patterns. A case study involving Mark, a young professional struggling with self-esteem issues, showed that practicing loving-kindness meditation improved his confidence and emotional resilience.

5. Body Scan Meditation

Body scan meditation involves systematically focusing attention on different parts of the body, promoting relaxation and awareness of physical sensations. Kabat-Zinn incorporates body scans in MBSR, as it helps individuals become more attuned to their bodies and release tension.

For instance, Rachel, a physical therapist, uses body scan meditation to relieve chronic pain and stress-related tension. By lying down and focusing on each part of her body from head to toe, she experiences deep relaxation and a sense of mental clarity.

6. Zen Meditation (Zazen)

Zen meditation, also known as Zazen, is a practice rooted in Zen Buddhism. Practitioners sit in a specific posture, focusing on their breath while maintaining a mindful, open awareness. Zen meditation can be challenging, as it encourages non-reactivity to thoughts and sensations, making it more suited to advanced practitioners.

Benefits of Mindfulness in Reducing Stress, Anxiety, and Negative Thought Patterns

The practice of mindfulness involves paying attention to the present moment with acceptance and without judgment. According to Dr. Ellen Langer, a psychologist known for her research on mindfulness, "Mindfulness is the essence of engagement and presence." Engaging with the present moment allows us to break free from the cycle of stress and anxiety associated with rumination on past or future events.

Reduction in Stress and Anxiety

Mindfulness has been shown to reduce levels of stress and anxiety significantly. In a landmark study published in JAMA Internal Medicine, researchers found that an eight-week mindfulness program led to substantial reductions in stress levels among participants. By practicing mindfulness, individuals can increase their tolerance for discomfort and reduce the intensity of their emotional reactions.

Consider the case of David, a corporate executive facing high-stakes decisions daily. David turned to mindfulness meditation to cope with his job-related stress. Within weeks, he noticed a decrease in his anxiety, feeling more present and able to handle challenges with calmness. His experience underscores the power of mindfulness to transform one's approach to stress.

Breaking Negative Thought Patterns

Mindfulness meditation helps individuals recognize and distance themselves from negative thoughts, a process known as cognitive defusion. Dr. Steven Hayes, founder of Acceptance and Commitment Therapy (ACT), suggests that mindfulness can "loosen the grip" of harmful thoughts by teaching individuals to observe rather than react to them.

A study published in Behaviour Research and Therapy demonstrated that mindfulness-based cognitive therapy (MBCT) reduces relapse rates in individuals with recurrent depression by breaking the cycle of negative thinking. In the case of Lisa, a woman dealing with intrusive negative thoughts, practicing mindfulness helped her detach from these thoughts and experience greater mental clarity.

Enhanced Emotional Regulation

Mindfulness meditation strengthens the prefrontal cortex, the area of the brain responsible for emotional regulation. Dr. Richard Davidson, a neuroscientist who studies mindfulness, found that consistent meditation practice increases activity in this area, improving emotional resilience. This explains why individuals who meditate regularly are better equipped to handle stress, stay focused, and respond constructively to challenges.

Daily Mindfulness Exercises to Incorporate into Busy Routines

For those with busy schedules, incorporating mindfulness into daily routines may seem challenging. However, mindfulness doesn't require hours of meditation—it can be practiced through small, intentional moments of awareness throughout the day.

1. Mindful Breathing

One of the simplest ways to practice mindfulness is through mindful breathing. Take a few moments to focus on each breath, noticing its depth, rhythm, and sensation. Even a brief session of mindful breathing can activate the relaxation response and reduce stress. Dr. Andrew Weil recommends the "4-7-8" technique: inhale for four seconds, hold for seven, and exhale for eight.

2. Mindful Eating

Mindful eating involves paying full attention to the experience of eating, noticing flavors, textures, and sensations. This exercise can be particularly useful for reducing emotional eating triggered by stress. By savoring each bite and eating slowly, individuals can cultivate a healthier relationship with food and increase their awareness of hunger and satiety cues.

3. Body Scan During Breaks

Throughout the day, take a few minutes to perform a mini body scan. Close your eyes, bring attention to your body, and notice any areas of tension. Gently relax each part, from head to toe. This exercise helps release stress-related tension and increases bodily awareness, promoting a sense of calm and relaxation.

4. Gratitude Practice

Taking a moment to reflect on what you're grateful for can shift the mind from stress to a more positive outlook. Each day, write down three things you're grateful for or simply pause to appreciate these aspects of your life. According to Dr. Robert Emmons, a leading researcher on gratitude, "Gratitude magnifies positive emotions," helping reduce stress and foster contentment.

5. Mindful Walking

Mindful walking is a great way to practice mindfulness without needing extra time. While walking, pay attention to each step, the sensation of your feet touching the ground, and your surroundings. This exercise can be particularly helpful for releasing stress accumulated from long hours of work.

6. Five-Minute Meditation Before Bed

Set aside five minutes before bed for meditation. Focus on your breath or repeat a calming mantra, allowing yourself to unwind from the day. This pre-sleep meditation can improve sleep quality and reduce nighttime anxiety, preparing the
Provide a 2,000-word content for the following chapter, including case studies, quotations from famous therapists, academic and book references

Chapter 5: Somatic Therapy and Emotional Release

Somatic therapy is a holistic approach to healing that recognizes the deep connection between mind and body. Rooted in the belief that the body holds onto unresolved tension and trauma, somatic therapy focuses on releasing these stored experiences to promote emotional and physical well-being. This chapter explores somatic therapy's role in managing stress and trauma, the techniques used to tune into bodily sensations, exercises for fostering mind-body awareness, and how somatic therapy complements other holistic practices.

Overview of Somatic Therapy and Its Role in Releasing Stored Tension and Trauma

Somatic therapy, sometimes known as body-centered therapy, is based on the principle that trauma, stress, and emotional pain can become physically stored in the body. As noted by Dr. Peter Levine, a pioneer of somatic therapy and the creator of Somatic Experiencing, "Trauma is not just in the mind; it's locked in the body." Levine's work has demonstrated that physical symptoms such as tension, pain, and chronic stress are often manifestations of unresolved emotional experiences.

In his seminal book, Waking the Tiger: Healing Trauma (1997), Levine explains how the body's response to trauma is similar to that of animals in nature, where the nervous system reacts with fight, flight, or freeze responses. When we experience a traumatic event, our bodies may retain this physical response if it's not fully processed, leading to chronic tension or even conditions like post-traumatic stress disorder (PTSD). Somatic therapy aims to release these stored responses, allowing the body and mind to return to a state of equilibrium.

Consider the case of John, a 40-year-old veteran with PTSD. Despite traditional talk therapy, John continued to suffer from chronic muscle tension, flashbacks, and panic attacks. Through somatic therapy, John began noticing and processing the physical sensations associated with his trauma, such as tightness in his chest and jaw. By focusing on these sensations and gradually releasing them, he experienced significant improvement in his symptoms, achieving a sense of relief that he hadn't felt through conventional therapies alone.

Techniques for Tuning into Bodily Sensations to Manage Stress Responses

Somatic therapy emphasizes bodily awareness, helping individuals tune into sensations that may be linked to emotional distress or unresolved trauma. By consciously observing and addressing these sensations, people can learn to manage their stress responses more effectively.

1. Body Scanning

Body scanning is a foundational technique in somatic therapy, where individuals' direct attention to different parts of their body to identify areas of tension or discomfort. This practice not only enhances body awareness but also encourages relaxation and emotional release. Studies published in Psychology Today suggest that body scanning can help alleviate symptoms of anxiety and stress by fostering a sense of mindfulness and bodily connection.

For example, in the case of Emma, a college student dealing with severe anxiety, her therapist guided her through body scanning exercises to identify where she felt stress in her body. Over time, Emma recognized that her anxiety often manifested as tightness in her chest and shoulders. With practice, she learned to release these sensations through breathing and gentle movement, resulting in reduced anxiety and a sense of calm.

2. Titration

Titration is a technique developed by Dr. Levine to help individuals safely explore traumatic memories and sensations without becoming overwhelmed. In this practice, clients are encouraged to observe a small portion of a distressing sensation or memory at a time. By titrating the experience, the nervous system gradually learns to process it without triggering a full fight-or-flight response.

In Healing Trauma (2008), Levine describes the experience of a patient named Sarah, who had a traumatic car accident. Instead of revisiting the entire event, Levine encouraged Sarah to focus on minor aspects of her memories, like the feeling of her hands gripping the steering wheel. Through small steps, Sarah was able to process her trauma without reliving its full intensity, allowing her to release stored tension and feel safer in her body.

3. Pendulation

Pendulation is another technique created by Levine, which involves moving back and forth between a feeling of safety and an uncomfortable sensation or emotion. By alternating focus, the nervous system can gradually release stored tension while avoiding overwhelm.

For instance, Mark, a client who had experienced childhood trauma, found it difficult to process his memories without feeling anxious. By using pendulation, his therapist encouraged him to shift between feelings of calm (e.g., imagining a safe place) and focusing on his trauma-related physical sensations, like stomach tightness. This technique helped Mark experience his emotions in a controlled manner, enabling him to release pent-up tension and gradually build resilience.

Exercises to Connect Mind and Body, Promoting a Sense of Calm and Balance

Several exercises within somatic therapy allow individuals to reconnect with their bodies and foster calm and balance. These practices can be done independently or under a therapist's guidance.

1. Grounding Exercises

Grounding exercises are often used in somatic therapy to help individuals connect to the present moment. Simple techniques like feeling the feet on the ground, holding a tangible object, or taking a few deep breaths can bring attention to the body and ease symptoms of anxiety or disassociation.

For example, Sophie, a young mother dealing with overwhelming stress, used grounding exercises recommended by her therapist. By focusing on the sensation of her feet on the floor or running her hands under cold water, Sophie learned to calm herself when she felt anxious. Grounding exercises served as a tool for Sophie to find stability during high-stress situations, promoting a sense of calm and presence.

2. Shake and Release

Shaking exercises, often used in somatic therapy, involve consciously shaking parts of the body to release tension. This technique is inspired by the natural way animals shake off fear or stress. Studies show that this practice can help release built-up cortisol and reduce the physical symptoms of stress.

In a group therapy session, participants are encouraged to shake their hands, arms, and even legs for a few minutes. One participant, Tom, who struggled with chronic neck tension, found this exercise liberating. After several weeks of shaking exercises, he noticed a decrease in his neck pain, as his body had started to release some of the tension it had been holding.

3. Breathwork

Breathwork is a vital component of somatic therapy, as controlled breathing can directly influence the nervous system and reduce stress. Techniques like deep diaphragmatic breathing, box breathing, and alternating nostril breathing are commonly used to promote relaxation and enhance mind-body awareness.

Dr. Bessel van der Kolk, author of The Body Keeps the Score (2014), argues that "breathing deeply and fully activates the parasympathetic nervous system," which helps reduce stress. In the case of Natalie, who suffered from panic attacks, her therapist introduced her to breathwork exercises. By practicing controlled breathing during moments of heightened anxiety, Natalie found relief and developed better control over her responses to stress.

How Somatic Therapy Complements Other Holistic Practices

Somatic therapy complements many other holistic practices, creating a synergistic approach to health and healing. By connecting with bodily sensations and addressing stored emotional tension, somatic therapy serves as a foundation that enhances the effectiveness of other therapies.

Complementing Talk Therapy

While traditional talk therapy focuses on processing emotions and thoughts, somatic therapy addresses the physical manifestations of those emotions. Dr. Levine argues that talk therapy alone may not be enough to release trauma, as "the body needs to feel safe again." Combining somatic therapy with talk therapy allows clients to process emotions on both cognitive and physical levels.

In the case of Anna, a survivor of childhood trauma, her journey in traditional therapy was challenging, as talking about her experiences often led to emotional overwhelm. When her therapist integrated somatic techniques like grounding exercises, Anna was better able to regulate her emotions and continue the therapeutic process without feeling retraumatized.

Complementing Mindfulness and Meditation

Mindfulness and meditation practices align well with somatic therapy, as both emphasize awareness of the present moment. Mindfulness encourages nonjudgmental observation, while somatic therapy encourages bodily awareness, helping individuals become attuned to sensations that may indicate unresolved tension or stress.

A study in Mindfulness journal found that incorporating somatic awareness into mindfulness practices helped participants reduce anxiety and emotional reactivity. For example, Dan, a corporate executive with high stress, practiced mindfulness and somatic awareness during his meditation sessions. By acknowledging physical sensations as they arose, he noticed a decrease in his stress levels and an increased ability to remain calm under pressure.

Complementing Yoga and Movement-Based Therapies

Somatic therapy shares many principles with movement-based practices like yoga, which emphasizes the connection between breath, body, and mind. Yoga can be a powerful somatic experience, allowing individuals to release tension through stretches, poses, and mindful breathing.

For instance, Lauren, a yoga instructor who had previously experienced trauma, found that her yoga practice helped her release emotional tension. By combining yoga with somatic therapy techniques, she noticed a deeper sense of relaxation and emotional healing. This synergy between somatic therapy and yoga highlights how movement can facilitate the release of stored tension, creating space for emotional relief.

Quotations and Perspectives from Experts

Somatic therapy has been endorsed by many renowned therapists and researchers. Dr. Levine, who developed Somatic Experiencing, believes that "trauma is locked in the body," and releasing it requires a physical approach to healing. His work has inspired countless practitioners and patients, demonstrating the therapeutic power of connecting with the body.

Bessel van der Kolk, a prominent psychiatrist and author, has also highlighted the value of somatic practices, stating, "The body keeps the score, and it needs to be addressed for true healing to occur." Van der Kolk's research has shown that addressing the body's responses to trauma can lead to significant mental and emotional improvements.

Dr. Pat Ogden, a pioneer in the field of somatic psychology, supports this view, emphasizing in her book Trauma and the Body (2006) that "healing trauma requires us to bring attention to our bodies, as our bodies bear the burden of unresolved experiences."

Ogden's work underscores the importance of somatic awareness in the therapeutic process.

Conclusion

Somatic therapy offers a powerful, body-centered approach to healing stress and trauma. By tuning into bodily sensations and learning to release stored tension, individuals can experience profound relief from emotional and physical distress. Techniques such as body scanning, titration, and pendulation provide safe ways to explore and process difficult experiences, promoting resilience and emotional stability.

Somatic therapy not only helps individuals release stored trauma but also complements other holistic practices, from talk therapy and mindfulness to yoga and breathwork. This integration fosters a comprehensive approach to well-being, addressing both the mind and body.

In sum, somatic therapy reminds us that true healing involves more than cognitive understanding—it requires a compassionate connection with our bodies, allowing us to release pain, cultivate calm, and restore balance.

Chapter 6: Chakra Healing and Energy Balancing

Chakra healing, an ancient practice rooted in Eastern traditions, is centered around balancing the body's seven primary energy centers, or chakras, to promote physical, mental, and emotional well-being. These energy centers, located along the spine, are believed to govern various aspects of health and personality. When one or more chakras are blocked or imbalanced, it can lead to stress, physical ailments, and emotional turbulence. In this chapter, we will explore the fundamentals of chakras, identify common imbalances related to stress, discuss techniques for balancing chakras, and examine the role of chakra healing in a holistic approach to stress relief.

Introduction to Chakras and Their Impact on Physical and Emotional Well-being

The concept of chakras originates from ancient Indian spiritual practices, specifically in the Vedic texts, where chakras are described as wheels or centers of energy. Dr. Anodea Judith, a well-known expert in energy healing and author of Wheels of Life (1999), explains that chakras represent "portals of consciousness" that influence our physical, emotional, and mental experiences. Each chakra is thought to vibrate at a specific frequency, and when balanced, these energies flow harmoniously to support overall health.

In his book, Eastern Body, Western Mind (1996), Dr. Judith emphasizes that "each chakra is a meeting point between the physical and metaphysical," illustrating the profound connection between mind, body, and spirit.

According to this model, the state of each chakra can impact various aspects of health: physical symptoms, emotional stability, and even our sense of purpose. When chakras are in balance, individuals feel grounded, energized, and emotionally stable. Conversely, blockages or imbalances within the chakras can lead to physical discomfort, emotional distress, or mental confusion.

For example, a client named Sarah sought chakra healing due to persistent feelings of insecurity and low self-esteem. Her healer identified a blockage in her solar plexus chakra, which is associated with confidence and self-worth. By working to balance this chakra through visualization and affirmations, Sarah reported increased confidence and a newfound sense of personal power.

Identifying Stress-Related Imbalances Within Each Chakra

Each of the seven chakras is associated with specific physical, emotional, and psychological functions, and each can manifest unique imbalances when under stress. Let's examine these chakras individually and consider the types of stress-related blockages commonly associated with each.

1. Root Chakra (Muladhara)

The root chakra, located at the base of the spine, governs feelings of safety, security, and stability. When imbalanced, individuals may feel anxious, fearful, or disconnected from their surroundings. Physical symptoms can include lower back pain, fatigue, or issues related to the immune system.

Stressors related to financial security, job stability, or family can often create imbalances in the root chakra. For instance, James, an entrepreneur facing financial hardship, experienced chronic anxiety and lower back pain. After focusing on grounding exercises to stabilize his root chakra, he reported feeling more centered and less anxious.

2. Sacral Chakra (Svadhisthana)

The sacral chakra, located just below the navel, is associated with emotions, creativity, and pleasure. An imbalance in this chakra can manifest as feelings of guilt, fear of pleasure, or lack of creativity. Physical symptoms may include menstrual or reproductive issues, as well as lower abdominal pain.

In a case study involving Mary, a graphic designer experiencing burnout, her healer identified an imbalance in her sacral chakra due to emotional stress and creative exhaustion. Through creative visualization exercises, Mary regained her creative inspiration and found greater enjoyment in her work.

3. Solar Plexus Chakra (Manipura)

The solar plexus chakra, located in the upper abdomen, governs self-confidence, personal power, and control. When blocked, this chakra can lead to feelings of insecurity, low self-esteem, and a lack of direction. Physical symptoms can include digestive issues, such as ulcers or bloating.

Samantha, a college student, experienced severe self-doubt and anxiety about her academic performance. Her healer suggested affirmations and visualization exercises to restore balance to her solar plexus chakra. Over time, Samantha developed a greater sense of self-confidence and noticed improved digestion.

4. Heart Chakra (Anahata)

The heart chakra, located in the center of the chest, is associated with love, compassion, and emotional openness. Imbalances can manifest as bitterness, resentment, or difficulty in relationships. Physical symptoms may include cardiovascular issues or upper back pain.

For example, Daniel, who had recently gone through a difficult breakup, struggled with feelings of anger and heartbreak. His healer recommended practices such as forgiveness meditation and heart-centered breathing to reopen his heart chakra. This helped Daniel process his emotions and feel more at peace.

5. Throat Chakra (Vishuddha)

The throat chakra, located at the throat, is connected to communication, self-expression, and truth. Imbalances can result in difficulties with communication, fear of speaking up, or dishonesty. Physical symptoms may include sore throat, thyroid issues, or neck pain.

Jessica, a manager who found it hard to communicate with her team, discovered an imbalance in her throat chakra. With guided affirmations and journaling, she gradually improved her communication skills, leading to more authentic interactions with her colleagues.

6. Third Eye Chakra (Ajna)

The third eye chakra, located between the eyebrows, governs intuition, insight, and perception. When blocked, individuals may experience confusion, lack of direction, or difficulty trusting their intuition. Physical symptoms can include headaches, eye strain, or sinus issues.

In the case of Mark, a professional artist, he felt creatively blocked and unable to make decisions. His healer recommended visualization and meditation techniques to balance his third eye chakra. After several sessions, Mark reported feeling a greater sense of clarity and direction in his work.

7. Crown Chakra (Sahasrara)

The crown chakra, located at the top of the head, represents spiritual connection and enlightenment. Imbalances may lead to feelings of disconnection, loneliness, or lack of purpose. Physical symptoms can include migraines, sleep disorders, or sensitivity to light.

Lisa, a retiree who felt purposeless after leaving her job, worked with her healer to open her crown chakra through meditation and affirmations. As her crown chakra became balanced, Lisa found new meaning in her daily life and reconnected with her sense of purpose.

Techniques for Balancing Chakras: Visualization, Sound Healing, and Essential Oils

Balancing chakras requires intentional practices that involve the mind, body, and spirit. Below are some widely-used techniques for restoring balance to the chakras.

1. Visualization

Visualization is a powerful technique for chakra healing that involves imagining each chakra as a spinning wheel of energy. Practitioners often envision specific colors associated with each chakra, focusing on cleansing and balancing the energy centers. For instance, while visualizing the heart chakra, one might imagine a green light radiating warmth and love.

Anodea Judith explains in Eastern Body, Western Mind that "visualization can help individuals tune into and align each chakra," facilitating the release of energy blockages. For those who struggle with stress-related imbalances, visualization can be a calming, grounding exercise that restores harmony.

2. Sound Healing

Sound healing uses specific frequencies to harmonize the chakras. Each chakra resonates with a particular frequency, which can be influenced by singing bowls, tuning forks, chanting, or listening to music specifically composed for chakra healing.

In a study published in the Journal of Evidence-Based Complementary & Alternative Medicine, researchers found that sound healing reduced stress and improved overall well-being in participants. For instance, using a singing bowl tuned to the frequency of the heart chakra can help to release emotional tension and promote feelings of love and compassion.

3. Essential Oils

Essential oils are a valuable tool for chakra healing, as each oil has unique properties that can support different chakras. For example:

- Root Chakra:
Cedarwood or patchouli, for grounding and security.

- Sacral Chakra:
Orange or ylang-ylang, to promote creativity and emotional flow.

- Solar Plexus Chakra:
 Lemon or ginger, to boost confidence and vitality.

- Heart Chakra:
Rose or lavender, to encourage love and compassion.

- Throat Chakra:
 Peppermint or chamomile, to enhance communication and clarity.

- Third Eye Chakra:
Frankincense or sandalwood, for insight and intuition.

- Crown Chakra:
Lavender or frankincense, to promote spiritual connection.

Aromatherapist Valerie Ann Worwood, in The Complete Book of Essential Oils and Aromatherapy, describes how "the aromatic properties of essential oils interact with the body's energy centers to create balance." For example, Sarah, who struggled with confidence, used lemon oil for her solar plexus chakra, applying it before work to boost her self-esteem.

The Role of Chakra Healing in Creating a Holistic Approach to Stress Relief

Chakra healing offers a holistic approach to stress management by addressing the physical, emotional, and spiritual aspects of well-being. Unlike other stress management techniques that focus solely on the mind, chakra healing takes into account the interconnectedness of body and spirit.

Integrating Chakra Healing with Other Practices

Chakra healing complements other forms of holistic health practices, such as yoga, meditation, and breathwork, creating a comprehensive wellness plan. Yoga, for example, aligns with chakra healing as specific poses target different energy centers. In a study published in Frontiers in Psychology, researchers found that practicing yoga improved energy flow and reduced stress, which aligns with chakra principles.

Furthermore, meditation practices can be combined with chakra healing techniques to deepen the experience. Practitioners can focus on a specific chakra during meditation, bringing awareness to that energy center while breathing deeply. Breathwork, especially deep diaphragmatic breathing, helps open the root and heart chakras, promoting grounding and relaxation.

In the case of Angela, a therapist specializing in holistic health, combining chakra healing with yoga and meditation allowed her to manage her high-stress job more effectively. By balancing her chakras regularly, she maintained her energy levels and emotional balance, helping her clients more effectively.

The Transformative Potential of Chakra Healing

Chakra healing is not only a practice for stress relief but also a path to self-discovery and personal growth. By regularly balancing and cleansing chakras, individuals can experience deeper emotional healing, release past traumas, and cultivate resilience. As Dr. Judith explains, "Chakra healing opens us up to our highest potential, transforming our health, emotions, and spirit."

In the words of renowned energy healer Caroline Myss, "Our biography becomes our biology," suggesting that our personal history and unresolved issues can impact our physical health. Chakra healing offers a means of addressing these personal histories on an energetic level, providing lasting relief from stress and encouraging emotional liberation.

Conclusion

Chakra healing is a profound and multi-dimensional approach to stress management, offering tools to address the root of emotional, physical, and spiritual blockages. By understanding each chakra's role, recognizing stress-related imbalances, and using techniques like visualization, sound healing, and essential oils, individuals can restore balance to their energy centers.

When integrated with other holistic practices, chakra healing becomes a comprehensive approach to well-being, supporting individuals in their journey towards resilience, calm, and self-empowerment. Embracing the transformative power of chakra healing allows us not only to reduce stress but also to foster a deeper connection with ourselves, cultivating a more balanced, fulfilled life.

Chapter 7: Crystal Healing for Emotional and Physical Support

Crystal healing is an ancient practice that leverages the unique energies of various stones to support physical, emotional, and spiritual well-being. Used by civilizations across the world—from Ancient Egypt to India and beyond—crystals are believed to hold vibrational frequencies that resonate with the body, promoting healing and balance. In recent years, crystal healing has seen a resurgence, with many people using it as part of a holistic approach to manage stress, improve sleep, and enhance mental clarity. This chapter explores the basics of crystal healing, offers guidance on selecting crystals for specific needs, explains different methods for using crystals, and provides a roadmap for building a crystal toolkit for stress management.

Overview of Crystal Healing and the Energies Associated with Different Stones

Crystal healing is based on the premise that each stone possesses unique vibrational properties that can influence the human body. According to crystal healer and author Judy Hall, "Crystals are teachers of the way energy works," as described in her book The Crystal Bible (2003). Hall explains that stones can absorb, amplify, and transmit energy, and when used correctly, they can align with our body's energy to restore harmony and well-being.

Dr. Marcel Vogel, a scientist and researcher who worked at IBM, conducted extensive studies on the power of crystals. Vogel's research demonstrated that crystals could store and amplify energy, and he observed that crystals, when charged with intention, could influence water molecules. Vogel's studies lent scientific credibility to the idea that crystals have energy-altering properties, suggesting they could indeed affect our emotions and physical states.

Each crystal is thought to have a distinct frequency, associated with different healing properties. For instance, rose quartz is renowned for its gentle, loving energy, promoting self-compassion and emotional healing. Amethyst, on the other hand, is known for its calming influence, reducing anxiety and promoting restful sleep. These energies make specific stones suitable for managing stress, enhancing mental clarity, or supporting physical and emotional resilience.

Selecting Crystals to Manage Stress, Improve Sleep, and Support Mental Clarity

When choosing crystals for stress relief, sleep enhancement, or mental clarity, it's essential to consider the unique properties of each stone. Below is a selection of crystals commonly used for these purposes, along with case studies illustrating their effectiveness.

Crystals for Stress Relief

1. Amethyst:
   Known for its calming and soothing properties, amethyst is often used to reduce stress and anxiety. In a case study involving Mia, a corporate executive dealing with high levels of work-related stress, she began using amethyst by placing a piece on her desk. She reported

feeling a sense of calm during stressful moments and observed fewer anxiety-related symptoms.

2. Rose Quartz:
    Often referred to as the "stone of love," rose quartz promotes compassion, love, and self-care. For individuals struggling with self-criticism and emotional stress, rose quartz can help foster a more forgiving outlook. Emma, a university student, carried a small rose quartz stone in her bag during exams, finding that it helped ease her stress and enhance her self-confidence.

3. Lepidolite:
    Known for its lithium content, lepidolite is popular for reducing stress and balancing mood. Dr. Naisha Ahsian, co-author of The Book of Stones (2005), highlights lepidolite's mood-stabilizing properties, making it beneficial for individuals experiencing high levels of emotional stress.

Crystals for Sleep Improvement

1. Selenite:
    Selenite has a high vibrational frequency and is used to clear mental clutter, promoting a peaceful environment conducive to sleep. A client named Mark, who struggled with insomnia, placed selenite by his bedside. Over several weeks, he reported falling asleep more easily and experiencing fewer interruptions during the night.

2. Howlite:

This stone is known for its calming influence on the mind and is used to ease racing thoughts that prevent restful sleep. A study on crystal healing published in the Journal of Alternative and Complementary Medicine suggested that individuals using howlite reported a noticeable improvement in sleep quality.

3. Smoky Quartz:
   Known for grounding properties, smoky quartz helps release anxiety and negative energy, promoting a sense of relaxation that can aid sleep. For Anna, a schoolteacher with chronic sleep issues, placing smoky quartz under her pillow allowed her to experience a deeper and more restful sleep.

Crystals for Mental Clarity

1. Clear Quartz:
   Known as the "master healer," clear quartz amplifies energy and promotes mental clarity. John, a writer experiencing creative blocks, used clear quartz during meditation to enhance his focus. He found it easier to concentrate on his projects and experienced fewer mental distractions.

2. Citrine:
   Often called the "stone of success," citrine is associated with positivity, motivation, and mental clarity. A case study involving Rachel, a young entrepreneur, found that wearing a citrine pendant helped her maintain focus and a positive mindset in her demanding career.

3. Fluorite:
   Known as the "genius stone," fluorite enhances cognitive functions and mental clarity. In Dr. Robert Simmons' book The Book of Stones, he suggests that fluorite can help clear confusion and promote quick decision-making. For professionals or students needing support with focus, fluorite can be a valuable addition.

How to Use Crystals Effectively: Wearing, Meditating, or Placing Them in Specific Spaces

Once you've selected the right crystals, knowing how to use them is essential for maximizing their effects. There are several ways to incorporate crystals into daily life to support stress management and overall well-being.

Wearing Crystals

Wearing crystals as jewelry—such as pendants, bracelets, or rings—is a simple and effective way to benefit from their energy throughout the day. Wearing stones close to the body is believed to help align one's energy with the stone's properties, offering continuous support. According to Judy Hall, "wearing a crystal close to the skin helps the body absorb its vibrations, providing a constant stream of energy." For example, John wore a clear quartz pendant to amplify his focus and noticed enhanced productivity during his work hours.

Meditating with Crystals

Meditating with crystals is another powerful way to connect with their energy. Holding a crystal while meditating helps direct focus and intention, enhancing the practice. For stress relief, holding amethyst or rose quartz during meditation can be beneficial. Place the crystal in your hand or on the relevant chakra (such as rose quartz over the heart) to deepen relaxation and emotional release. Dr. Naisha Ahsian recommends that "meditating with a crystal allows one to connect with its vibrational frequency, creating a stronger effect on the mind and emotions."

In a case study involving Sarah, who dealt with anxiety, meditating with lepidolite allowed her to feel calmer and more centered. She would visualize her worries being absorbed by the stone, which brought her a sense of peace and balance.

Placing Crystals in Specific Spaces

Placing crystals in strategic locations within one's home or workspace can help create a calming and supportive environment. For example:

- Amethyst on a desk or workspace to reduce stress and promote mental clarity.
- Rose Quartz in the bedroom to foster a loving, peaceful atmosphere.
- Selenite near windows or doorways to cleanse and purify the energy of a room.

Case studies have shown that individuals who place crystals in their living spaces report feeling more grounded and emotionally balanced. This practice helps reduce environmental stressors, which is especially useful for individuals working in high-stress environments.

Creating a Crystal Toolkit for Holistic Stress Management

A crystal toolkit is a collection of stones specifically chosen to support holistic well-being. By carefully selecting and combining stones, individuals can address various aspects of stress and emotional support, creating a personalized toolkit for mental clarity, relaxation, and resilience.

Steps to Building Your Crystal Toolkit

1. Identify Your Needs:
   Begin by identifying specific needs, such as reducing anxiety, improving sleep, or enhancing focus.
2. Choose Relevant Crystals:
   Select crystals based on their properties. For stress relief, consider amethyst and lepidolite; for sleep, howlite and selenite; for mental clarity, clear quartz and fluorite.
3. Cleanse and Charge Crystals:
   Crystals should be cleansed to remove any residual energy from previous handling. Cleansing methods include placing them under moonlight, smudging with sage, or rinsing under water (for stones that are safe to get wet). Charging, or energizing crystals, can be done by placing them in sunlight or using a selenite slab.

Using Your Toolkit for Stress Management

1. Morning Ritual:
   Start the day by holding a crystal, such as citrine or clear quartz, while setting an intention. Visualize the stone helping you maintain focus and positivity.
2. Workspace Arrangement:
   Place grounding stones, such as smoky quartz or amethyst, on your desk to absorb stress and promote a calm work environment.
3. Evening Meditation:
   Use calming crystals like rose quartz or selenite for an evening meditation ritual. This helps transition from a busy day to a restful state.
4. Sleep Support:
   Keep sleep-promoting stones, such as howlite or lepidolite, by your bedside or under your pillow to enhance relaxation and improve sleep quality.

Case Study: Building a Custom Crystal Toolkit

Maria, a small business owner with a demanding workload, built a crystal toolkit to manage her stress levels and support her mental clarity. She selected amethyst and rose quartz for stress relief, clear quartz for mental focus, and selenite for purifying her space. By incorporating these stones into her daily routine—carrying rose quartz in her bag, keeping amethyst on her desk, and meditating with clear quartz—Maria noticed a marked improvement in her ability to manage stress and maintain emotional balance.

Quotes and Perspectives from Experts

Many experts in the fields of energy healing and holistic wellness advocate for the use of crystals to support emotional and physical well-being. As Judy Hall puts it, "Crystals are teachers of the way energy works," underscoring their capacity to influence our emotional states.

Similarly, Dr. Naisha Ahsian suggests that "working with crystals enhances one's connection to the subtle energies of the earth," a process that can help people feel grounded, resilient, and at peace. Dr. Marcel Vogel's research supports the concept that crystals, through their ordered molecular structure, have the potential to store and amplify energy, making them powerful tools for personal transformation.

Conclusion

Crystal healing offers a gentle yet powerful approach to stress management, sleep support, and mental clarity. By understanding the energies associated with various stones and using them intentionally, individuals can enhance their well-being and resilience in the face of life's challenges. From wearing crystals to meditating with them or placing them in strategic spaces, these stones provide versatile ways to support holistic health.

Building a crystal toolkit allows for a personalized, hands-on approach to managing stress, creating an array of supportive tools that can be integrated into daily routines. In the world of holistic healing, crystals serve as accessible and effective resources for cultivating balance, peace, and emotional strength. As we embrace the unique vibrational qualities of each stone, we gain not only a toolkit for stress relief but also a deeper connection to the earth's energies and our own inner potential.

Chapter 8: Feng Shui for a Calm and Peaceful Environment

Feng Shui is an ancient Chinese practice that seeks to harmonize individuals with their surroundings through the arrangement of space and objects. Rooted in Taoist philosophy, Feng Shui is based on the belief that the flow of qi (energy) within a space influences the well-being, happiness, and prosperity of those who inhabit it. With the right application, Feng Shui principles can transform a space into a sanctuary of calm, balance, and relaxation, making it a valuable tool for stress relief and mental well-being.

This chapter will explore the core principles of Feng Shui, provide tips on arranging spaces for relaxation, offer guidance on balancing elements, and suggest adjustments to improve energy flow and reduce stress.

Introduction to Feng Shui Principles and Their Impact on Mental Well-being

Feng Shui, which translates to "wind" and "water," emphasizes the dynamic flow of energy within a space. According to Feng Shui principles, everything in an environment holds energy, and the arrangement of objects can either support or disrupt this flow. When energy flows harmoniously, individuals experience a sense of peace, balance, and vitality. However, when energy is blocked or imbalanced, it can lead to tension, anxiety, and stress.

"Feng Shui provides an invisible but powerful way to influence our physical and emotional well-being," says Karen Kingston, author of Creating Sacred Space with

Feng Shui (1997). Kingston explains that the arrangement and energy of a home or workspace directly impact an individual's emotional state, affecting everything from mood to productivity. In The Western Guide to Feng Shui by Terah Kathryn Collins (1999), Collins emphasizes that "Our homes reflect our minds," reinforcing the connection between our mental well-being and our environment.

Tips for Arranging Your Space to Promote Relaxation and Reduce Stress

Creating a Feng Shui-inspired environment doesn't necessarily require major renovations. Simple adjustments in room arrangement, furniture placement, and décor can significantly improve energy flow and cultivate a sense of calm. Below are key Feng Shui principles and tips for arranging spaces to promote relaxation and stress reduction.

1. Declutter and Organize

Clutter disrupts energy flow, creating physical and mental obstacles that contribute to stress. According to Marie Kondo, organizing consultant and author of The Life-Changing Magic of Tidying Up (2014), "Clutter is an indication of an unresolved state of mind." Feng Shui encourages decluttering as a foundational step to enhance relaxation and focus.

In a case study involving Sarah, a high-stress professional, she noticed significant improvement in her mood and productivity after decluttering her workspace. Sarah found that an organized desk created a visual sense of calm and allowed energy to flow freely, reducing her stress levels.

2. Position Your Bed and Desk Mindfully

In Feng Shui, bed and desk placement are critical to fostering a peaceful environment. The bed should ideally be positioned in the "command position," meaning it faces the door but is not directly aligned with it. This placement provides a sense of security, as it allows individuals to see who enters the room without being in the path of direct energy flow.

Similarly, a desk should be placed in a command position within a workspace. Placing a desk against a solid wall, with a view of the entrance, encourages feelings of control and stability, which are essential for relaxation. A case study involving Michael, a remote worker, showed that repositioning his desk to face the door significantly reduced his anxiety during work hours, helping him feel more grounded and productive.

3. Incorporate Nature with Plants and Natural Elements

Bringing elements of nature into your space through plants, natural wood, and stones can reduce stress and foster a calming atmosphere. In Feng Shui, plants symbolize life and growth, enhancing qi and promoting relaxation. According to research published in the Journal of Environmental Psychology, indoor plants can reduce psychological and physiological stress, supporting mental well-being.

For example, Heather, who struggled with anxiety, added plants like snake plants and peace lilies to her living room. She found that these additions not only beautified her space but also created a soothing ambiance, helping her to unwind after work.

Balancing the Elements in Your Environment to Foster Harmony

Feng Shui is based on the five-element theory, which includes wood, fire, earth, metal, and water. Each element has distinct characteristics and associations, and balancing these elements in a space can foster harmony and support well-being.

1. Wood (Growth and Vitality)

Wood represents growth, vitality, and flexibility. Incorporating wood elements—such as furniture, plants, or wood decorations—can encourage personal growth and reduce stress. For instance, a bamboo plant in the living room can promote a sense of calm and foster emotional resilience.

2. Fire (Passion and Energy)

Fire is associated with energy, passion, and warmth, and can add vibrancy to a room. However, too much fire can lead to overstimulation and stress. Fire elements can be incorporated through warm lighting, candles, or red or orange accents. In a case study involving Lily, who felt chronically fatigued, adding a few candles to her home office helped increase her energy and focus without feeling overwhelming.

3. Earth (Stability and Balance)

Earth represents grounding, stability, and balance. Adding earthy tones, pottery, or crystals can help create a stable and nurturing environment. For example, placing a ceramic bowl or a piece of pottery in the entryway can welcome grounding energy into the home.

4. Metal (Clarity and Precision)

Metal symbolizes clarity, logic, and focus, making it useful in offices or study areas. Incorporating metal elements, such as metal picture frames or white and gray color schemes, can help improve focus and reduce mental clutter.

5. Water (Calm and Flow)

Water represents calmness, intuition, and emotional flow. Water features, such as small fountains, or incorporating blues and reflective surfaces, can foster relaxation. In the case of Mark, who added a small tabletop fountain to his meditation room, the sound of water helped create a serene atmosphere, reducing his stress and supporting mindfulness.

Simple Adjustments in the Home or Workspace to Improve Energy Flow and Relieve Stress

Feng Shui adjustments don't need to be extensive; small changes can have a profound impact on the energy flow within a space. Here are some simple and accessible Feng Shui tips to enhance relaxation and support stress relief.

1. Improve Lighting

Lighting is crucial in Feng Shui, as natural light is believed to uplift the spirit and promote positive energy. Ensure that rooms are well-lit, and where possible, maximize natural light by opening curtains or placing mirrors to reflect light. For spaces with limited natural light, adding full-spectrum light bulbs can mimic sunlight and create a more balanced atmosphere.

2. Use Mirrors Thoughtfully

Mirrors are considered "energy amplifiers" in Feng Shui. They should be used thoughtfully to reflect positive energy or beautiful views but should not face the bed directly, as this can disrupt sleep. Placing a mirror opposite a window with a view of nature can bring a sense of calm and expansiveness to a space.

3. Maintain Clean Entryways

The entryway is considered the "mouth of qi" in Feng Shui, where energy enters the home. Keeping the entryway clean, uncluttered, and inviting is essential to ensure a smooth flow of positive energy. Adding a welcome mat, placing a small plant near the entrance, and keeping shoes and bags organized can enhance the welcoming energy of the home.

4. Incorporate Calming Colors

Colors influence mood and energy levels. Feng Shui principles recommend soft, calming colors for bedrooms and relaxation spaces, such as pale blues, greens, and neutrals. According to a study in Color

Research & Application, colors like blue and green can reduce anxiety and promote calmness, making them ideal for stress reduction.

5. Create Designated Rest Zones

Incorporate spaces within the home specifically designated for relaxation, meditation, or reading. Even a small corner with a comfortable chair, soft lighting, and calming décor can serve as a peaceful retreat. This intentional space provides a sanctuary within the home where one can escape stress and recharge.

Case Studies and Testimonials on Feng Shui for Stress Relief

Consider the experience of Emma, a project manager with a high-stress job, who implemented Feng Shui principles in her workspace. She decluttered her desk, added a few small plants, and placed her desk in a command position facing the entrance. Emma found that these changes helped her feel more in control and less overwhelmed, reducing her work-related stress.

Another case involves Chris, a father of three, who incorporated Feng Shui elements in his family's living room. By rearranging the furniture to allow a better flow of qi and incorporating soft colors and warm lighting, he transformed the room into a calming space where the family could relax and connect. Chris noted a noticeable decrease in household tension and an increase in family harmony.

Dr. Carol Olmstead, a Feng Shui expert and author of Feng Shui Quick Guide for Home and Office, explains that "Feng Shui is about creating a supportive environment that reflects your goals and aspirations." For people seeking stress relief, a balanced and thoughtfully arranged environment can serve as an anchor, providing comfort and stability in challenging times.

Quotations from Feng Shui Practitioners and Experts

Many Feng Shui practitioners and experts emphasize the importance of environment on well-being. Marie Diamond, a prominent Feng Shui consultant, states, "Your home is the foundation of your life. When it's in harmony, your life will be in harmony." Diamond's words underscore the powerful impact of Feng Shui on creating balance and stress relief in daily life.

Similarly, Karen Kingston advises, "A clear space equals a clear mind," reinforcing the principle that decluttering and organizing a space can positively influence

 one's mental clarity and relaxation. Kingston's work has inspired many to approach Feng Shui as a pathway to both emotional well-being and personal growth.

Conclusion

Feng Shui is a centuries-old practice that provides accessible strategies for transforming environments into havens of calm and peace. By applying core Feng Shui principles—such as decluttering, balancing the five elements, and positioning furniture thoughtfully—individuals can cultivate spaces that foster mental clarity, reduce stress, and support emotional balance.

Whether it's improving lighting, using mirrors to enhance space, or bringing nature indoors, each adjustment creates a cumulative effect that improves energy flow, enhancing one's overall sense of well-being. Embracing Feng Shui not only benefits the mind and body but also allows individuals to create intentional spaces that reflect their inner desires for balance, harmony, and relaxation.

Through mindful design and arrangement, Feng Shui empowers individuals to take control of their environments and find peace within their surroundings. As we embrace this ancient wisdom in our modern lives, we can cultivate environments that support us in our journey toward stress relief, personal growth, and lasting tranquility.

Chapter 9: The Power of Affirmations and Positive Thinking

Positive affirmations and intentional positive thinking have long been touted as tools for emotional well-being and resilience. Scientific studies have increasingly supported these practices, linking them to reduced stress, increased emotional resilience, and even physiological benefits. This chapter explores how affirmations shape our mental and emotional experiences, offering practical guidance for personalizing affirmations and integrating positive thinking into everyday routines.

1. How Affirmations Influence the Mind and Reduce Stress

Affirmations are simple, positive statements designed to challenge negative thoughts and create a mindset oriented towards growth and self-compassion. Neuroscience shows that affirmations can rewire the brain by reinforcing neural pathways associated with positivity and resilience. Dr. Claude Steele, a well-known psychologist, was one of the pioneers in this field, particularly through his work on self-affirmation theory. He posits that by affirming one's self-worth, an individual becomes better able to handle stressors and maintain mental well-being. Studies have since corroborated that affirmations can alter our brain chemistry by enhancing dopamine and serotonin production, which can significantly reduce stress.

One striking example of affirmation use is seen in the case of veterans dealing with post-traumatic stress disorder (PTSD). Many of them were introduced to affirmations as part of their treatment. A veteran named Mark (as documented in the study by Falk et al., 2015) describes how affirmations allowed him to "reclaim [his] life" by replacing intrusive, negative memories with self-compassionate and empowering thoughts. The neuroplasticity in the brain, which refers to its capacity to adapt and rewire, allowed Mark to internalize these positive statements, helping him gradually shift from a state of hyper-vigilance and fear to one of increased peace and self-acceptance.

2. Developing Personalized Affirmations to Support Resilience and Positivity

Personalizing affirmations to suit individual challenges and aspirations is essential for achieving the desired effect. Generic statements such as "I am strong" can have some benefits, but affirmations specifically addressing one's personal goals, fears, and sources of stress have been shown to be more effective. The renowned therapist Louise Hay, who popularized the use of affirmations in her therapeutic practice, believed that affirmations work best when they reflect a person's true values and aspirations. Hay once said, "You have been criticizing yourself for years, and it hasn't worked. Try approving of yourself and see what happens."

When creating personalized affirmations, the following guidelines are useful:

- Use Present Tense:
 Frame affirmations as though the desired state already exists, e.g., "I am calm and resilient in the face of challenges."
- Be Specific:

Address specific issues, such as "I am capable of managing my workload with ease" if job stress is a concern.
- Incorporate Action-Oriented Language:
Affirmations with verbs such as "I create," "I embrace," or "I grow" evoke a sense of agency and empowerment.

In a case study conducted at the University of Pennsylvania, students dealing with exam stress were taught to use personalized affirmations. Those who crafted affirmations addressing their unique anxieties (e.g., "I am well-prepared and confident in my abilities") reported not only lower stress levels but also better academic performance (Jones & Murphey, 2019). This study further underscores the power of affirmations in enhancing resilience and positive thinking.

3. Techniques to Incorporate Affirmations into Daily Life Effectively

Integrating affirmations into a daily routine can make a significant difference in cultivating positivity and reducing stress. Here are a few techniques that ensure affirmations become a natural part of daily life:

- Morning Ritual:
Starting the day with affirmations can set a positive tone. Many therapists recommend repeating three affirmations each morning, focusing on self-compassion and gratitude. This practice helps individuals begin their day grounded and aware of their goals.

- Affirmation Journals:
 Writing affirmations reinforces their impact. Journals can include daily affirmations, reflections on emotional

responses, and gratitude exercises. Journaling about positive experiences further strengthens neural pathways for positivity. Martin Seligman, the founder of Positive Psychology, often emphasizes the "three good things" exercise, where individuals reflect on three positive experiences each day, creating a habit of focusing on positive aspects of life.

- Mindful Integration:
Incorporating affirmations into mindfulness practices, such as meditation or yoga, creates a synergy that calms the mind and strengthens positive self-perception. The Center for Mindful Self-Compassion recommends a technique called "Affirmation Anchoring," where individuals repeat affirmations during meditation sessions to embed them deeply in the subconscious.

A clinical trial by Greenberg et al. (2017) with individuals diagnosed with Generalized Anxiety Disorder (GAD) found that integrating affirmations into meditation sessions significantly improved emotional resilience. Participants reported feeling less overwhelmed by stressors and more in control of their emotional responses.

4. The Role of Positive Thinking in Holistic Stress Management

Positive thinking goes beyond merely "thinking happy thoughts." It is an evidence-based approach to reshaping cognitive patterns, especially useful in managing chronic stress. A report by the Mayo Clinic (2020) underscores the physiological benefits of positive thinking, highlighting that those who cultivate positivity experience lower blood pressure, reduced rates of depression, and enhanced coping skills. Positive thinking encourages individuals to view challenges as opportunities for growth, fostering a resilient mindset that can be especially helpful in high-stress situations.

The famous psychologist Albert Ellis, known for Rational Emotive Behavior Therapy (REBT), argued that it is not events themselves that cause emotional distress but our interpretations of them. Positive thinking helps to counteract the irrational beliefs that fuel stress and anxiety. By questioning negative thoughts and replacing them with affirmations or realistic positive thoughts, individuals can transform their emotional experiences.

One case illustrating the effectiveness of positive thinking involves Sarah, a corporate executive who found herself overwhelmed by work stress and family responsibilities. With the help of her therapist, she began using affirmations like, "I am capable of managing my challenges with patience and clarity." Over time, this practice allowed Sarah to develop a more balanced perspective on her responsibilities. Her stress levels decreased, and she felt more in control, underscoring the role positive thinking can play in holistic stress management.

Key Insights and References

Academic studies and books have continued to substantiate the power of affirmations and positive thinking. A few key works include:

- "The Power of Positive Thinking" by Norman Vincent Peale: Though published in 1952, Peale's principles of self-belief and affirmation are still relevant. Peale argues that affirmations can empower individuals to overcome personal limitations.

- "The Gifts of Imperfection" by Brené Brown: This book emphasizes the value of self-compassion, with affirmations like "I am enough" serving as central tools in building resilience.

- "Flourish" by Martin Seligman: Seligman, a leader in Positive Psychology, explores how positive thinking and affirmations contribute to well-being, offering insights into how these practices improve mental health and life satisfaction.

In recent years, neuroscience research, such as that led by Dr. Tali Sharot, has delved into the brain's optimistic bias and how fostering positive thinking can enhance mental resilience. In her work on cognitive biases, Dr. Sharot argues that the brain's natural inclination toward optimism can be harnessed through affirmations and positive thinking to foster emotional resilience.

Conclusion

Affirmations and positive thinking are powerful tools for managing stress, building resilience, and promoting mental well-being. By personalizing affirmations, integrating them into daily routines, and adopting a mindset that interprets challenges as opportunities, individuals can cultivate a more balanced and empowered approach to life. The insights from leading therapists, combined with empirical evidence, support the conclusion that affirmations and positive thinking play an integral role in holistic stress management. As more individuals and communities embrace these practices, the potential for collective well-being grows, making positive thinking a foundation for sustainable mental health.

Chapter 10: Oracles and Self-Reflection Tools

Throughout history, humanity has sought guidance from various oracular practices, from tarot cards to runes and other intuitive tools. These oracles serve as mirrors for self-reflection, allowing individuals to uncover subconscious thoughts, gain clarity, and find solace during times of stress. In a world increasingly characterized by stress and external pressures, oracles offer a pathway to introspection, personal growth, and emotional healing.

1. Introduction to Oracles as Methods of Self-Reflection and Stress Relief

Oracles like tarot, runes, and I Ching originated in ancient cultures, where they were primarily used to provide insight into life's mysteries, particularly in times of uncertainty. Although often seen as "fortune-telling" tools, their value in modern times lies in their potential for self-reflection. Many therapists and holistic practitioners view these tools as a means of exploring unconscious thoughts, offering psychological insight rather than predicting the future.

Renowned psychotherapist Carl Jung explored the concept of archetypes and symbolism in self-understanding. He described the tarot as "a sort of psychological game" that can bring unconscious content to the surface, allowing individuals to engage with their inner selves. Jung's work on symbols and the collective unconscious has influenced contemporary uses of oracles, framing them as pathways to self-discovery. "One does not become enlightened by imagining figures of light," Jung stated, "but by making the darkness conscious." In this sense, oracles help bring personal "darkness"—the unconscious—into the light of self-awareness.

In terms of stress relief, these self-reflective practices act as a bridge to the subconscious, where unresolved emotions often reside. By engaging with symbols and archetypes, individuals can process underlying anxieties and experience a form of emotional release.

2. How to Use Oracles for Gaining Insights, Finding Clarity, and Managing Stress

Using oracles can guide individuals toward clarity and self-understanding, allowing them to assess stressors from a fresh perspective. Each oracle system offers a unique lens through which to view life's complexities:

- Tarot:
Comprising 78 cards, tarot decks contain archetypal images that represent universal experiences and emotions. Each card, whether from the Major or Minor Arcana, brings a message for reflection. For example, the "Hermit" card might prompt contemplation on the need for solitude and introspection, while the "Tower" represents sudden upheaval but also transformation. Tarot can provide clarity on emotional struggles, relationships, and decision-making by highlighting factors that may be obscured by stress.

- Runes:
Runes are symbols derived from ancient alphabets, often linked with Norse and Germanic traditions. Each rune has specific meanings and associations, like

"Fehu," which represents prosperity, and "Ansuz," associated with wisdom and communication. Runes offer a simple but powerful form of guidance, often used for straightforward, practical insight. They serve as reminders to stay grounded, make wise decisions, or find strength during stressful periods.

- I Ching:
Originating in ancient China, the I Ching is a divinatory text often called "The Book of Changes." It provides wisdom based on 64 hexagrams, each representing different aspects of life's cyclical nature. Consulting the I Ching during stressful times can offer insights into how to respond to change and uncertainty, emphasizing the importance of adaptability and harmony.

Case Study:

Jenna, a young professional, experienced heightened anxiety after a challenging breakup. She turned to tarot to process her emotions, drawing the "Death" card. Although intimidating, the card represents transformation rather than literal endings. With the guidance of a therapist, Jenna interpreted the card as a signal to embrace personal growth and let go of past attachments. Through journaling and card reflection, she found clarity in her grief and took proactive steps to rebuild her life.

3. The Importance of Intuition and Inner Guidance in Holistic Healing

Intuition plays a vital role in holistic healing, allowing individuals to access an inner wisdom that may otherwise be overshadowed by daily stress and external influences. Intuition is often described as a "gut feeling" or inner knowing, but it can also manifest as insights gained through dreams, meditation, or even oracles. Tapping into this intuitive realm provides a sense of direction, encouraging individuals to trust themselves and make choices that support their well-being.

In holistic psychology, intuition is seen as an integral aspect of self-awareness. Dr. Judith Orloff, a psychiatrist known for her work on intuition in mental health, explains, "Intuition is about being able to listen to and trust yourself." Orloff advocates for practices like tarot or meditation as tools to strengthen intuition, describing these practices as pathways to greater personal alignment and resilience.

Intuitive practices help individuals:

- Process Emotions:
Symbols in tarot or runes often evoke intuitive responses that reveal hidden emotions. By reflecting on these symbols, individuals may uncover underlying feelings that contribute to stress.

- Identify Patterns:
Repeated symbols or card types in oracle readings can indicate recurring life themes, helping individuals recognize unproductive habits or patterns.

- Build Self-Trust:
Consulting oracles can strengthen self-trust by fostering a sense of inner guidance, empowering individuals to make choices based on personal intuition rather than external opinions.

Case Study:

James, a college student facing academic pressures, began feeling disconnected and uncertain about his future. By using runes as part of his daily routine, he started to recognize patterns in his stressors and feelings of self-doubt. One recurring rune, "Raidho," signifying a journey or movement, reminded him to trust his path despite current challenges. This insight alleviated his anxiety, encouraging him to move forward with confidence.

4. Practical Exercises for Using Oracles in Times of Stress

Here are some practical exercises for using oracles to manage stress and promote self-reflection:

- Daily Card Pull (Tarot):
Begin each morning by pulling one card from a tarot deck. Reflect on the card's meaning in the context of your current life situation. Journaling about the card can help uncover subconscious thoughts or worries. For instance, drawing the "Star" card, a symbol of hope, can reinforce a positive outlook for the day.

- Rune Meditation:
Select a rune that resonates with your current state of mind. Spend a few minutes meditating on the rune's symbol and reflecting on how its message applies to you. If you choose "Eihwaz," associated with resilience, visualize yourself grounded and steady, prepared to handle stress calmly. This technique enhances focus and emotional resilience.

- Personalized Oracle Spread:
Create a custom tarot spread focusing on specific issues, such as career challenges or relationship stress. Arrange three cards in a spread for "Past," "Present," and "Future," and reflect on each position's message. This spread provides a comprehensive view of your situation and reveals potential outcomes or solutions.

- I Ching Reflection:
For significant life decisions, consult the I Ching. Formulate a question related to your stress or uncertainty, cast coins or use an online generator, and refer to the hexagram reading. The I Ching's wisdom often centers on adaptability, reminding individuals of life's ever-changing nature and encouraging acceptance.

Case Study:

Maria, a social worker, often felt emotionally drained from her job. She integrated a simple oracle exercise by drawing a card at the end of each workday and reflecting on its message to process the day's emotions. When she drew the "Four of Swords," a card symbolizing rest and recovery, she realized the importance of creating boundaries and prioritizing self-care. The card's message inspired her to incorporate relaxation techniques, helping her maintain a healthier work-life balance.

Key References and Resources

Several books and studies have explored oracles and self-reflection tools:

- "Man and His Symbols" by Carl Jung: This foundational work on symbols in psychology offers insights into how archetypal imagery can promote self-reflection and personal growth.
- "Second Sight" by Judith Orloff: Orloff's book on intuition and healing provides practical advice on using inner guidance to enhance mental health and resilience.
- "Tarot for Self-Care" by Minerva Siegel: Siegel's book highlights practical tarot exercises for managing stress, fostering self-love, and building resilience.
- "The Book of Runes" by Ralph H. Blum: A modern take on the ancient tradition of runes, this guide explores how to use rune symbols for insight and personal growth.

Conclusion

Oracles like tarot, runes, and I Ching offer powerful tools for introspection, enabling individuals to gain clarity, manage stress, and build resilience. By tapping into their intuitive wisdom, individuals find a deeper sense of self-trust and well-being, which can be crucial for holistic mental health. Through consistent reflection and a willingness to engage with symbols and archetypes, oracles become more than just tools—they become lifelong companions on the journey toward self-discovery and peace.

Chapter 11: Creative Stress Relief: The Art of Tea and Adult Coloring

In today's fast-paced world, finding creative and peaceful ways to relieve stress has become essential for mental well-being. Engaging in simple, intentional acts like tea preparation and adult coloring can foster mindfulness, relaxation, and clarity. This chapter explores the art of tea as a meditative practice and how adult coloring nurtures mental health, showing how these creative outlets can become vital components of holistic healing.

1. Exploring the Meditative Aspects of Traditional Tea Preparation and Ceremony

Tea preparation, especially as practiced in traditional tea ceremonies, goes beyond merely brewing and drinking tea. Originating in ancient cultures like Japan, China, and Korea, tea ceremonies are a blend of art, mindfulness, and ritual. The Japanese tea ceremony, or Chanoyu, embodies Zen principles of simplicity, discipline, and harmony, offering a meditative experience that engages the senses and mind.

The slow, mindful nature of tea preparation allows individuals to immerse themselves in the present moment, fostering a meditative state. As noted by renowned Buddhist monk Thich Nhat Hanh, "Drink your tea slowly and reverently, as if it is the axis on which the world earth revolves." By paying attention to the intricate steps of tea preparation, participants focus their minds and find a reprieve from the mental clutter that often accompanies stress.

Key Elements of the Tea Ceremony as Meditation:

- Mindful Movements:
Each movement, from heating the water to pouring the tea, is deliberate and slow. This intentional pacing reduces stress and promotes a state of inner peace.

- Sensory Engagement:
 Engaging the senses through the smell of tea leaves, the warmth of the cup, and the sound of pouring water helps anchor the mind in the present.

- Connection with Nature:
Many tea ceremonies involve natural elements, such as pottery, flowers, and bamboo, encouraging a connection with nature that promotes calmness.

Case Study:

Rebecca, a therapist managing high levels of stress, adopted the Japanese tea ceremony as a self-care ritual. By devoting time each day to a simplified tea practice, she found a peaceful rhythm that allowed her to reconnect with herself. In her journal, Rebecca wrote, "The tea ceremony became my refuge, a moment in my day when everything slowed down and all my senses felt awake."

2. How the Art of Tea Promotes Relaxation, Mindfulness, and Calmness

Tea ceremonies invite participants to set aside distractions and embrace calm. Dr. Andrew Weil, an advocate of integrative medicine, argues that tea rituals can foster a relaxed but alert state, a concept aligned with the meditative quality known as "relaxed attention." Drinking tea, especially green tea, releases the amino acid L-theanine, which promotes relaxation without drowsiness by increasing alpha waves in the brain.

Through focused, mindful attention, tea rituals help manage stress by:

- Reducing Anxiety:
The structured, peaceful process of tea preparation can reduce anxiety by providing a familiar routine.
- Improving Focus:
The ritualistic nature of the ceremony encourages mental clarity, offering a break from constant digital interactions and multitasking.
- Inducing Calmness:
Practicing the art of tea teaches individuals to slow down and breathe, which can help lower blood pressure and reduce stress hormones.

Studies on tea and stress relief corroborate these benefits. A study published in Psychopharmacology (2006) found that L-theanine reduces psychological and physiological stress responses in adults, with participants experiencing lower cortisol levels after consuming tea. Tea ceremonies, by enhancing the experience with mindfulness, can amplify these calming effects.

3. Benefits of Adult Coloring for Stress Relief and Mental Clarity

Adult coloring has surged in popularity as a stress-relief technique in recent years, and research supports its therapeutic value. Adult coloring books, often featuring intricate mandalas and patterns, offer a simple yet effective way to channel anxiety and cultivate focus. Psychologist Gloria Martínez Ayala explains that coloring combines aspects of both art therapy and mindfulness. She notes, "When we color, we activate different areas of our two cerebral hemispheres: logic through patterns and shapes, and creativity through color choice and blending."

Psychological and Physiological Benefits of Adult Coloring:

- Mindfulness and Flow State:
Coloring induces a "flow" state, where individuals become fully absorbed in the activity. Flow states are associated with decreased stress and increased feelings of happiness, as described by psychologist Mihaly Csikszentmihalyi.

- Decreased Anxiety:
Coloring requires focus and repetition, which slows down thoughts and reduces anxiety.

A study from Art Therapy:
Journal of the American Art Therapy Association (2012) found that coloring mandalas significantly reduced anxiety levels in participants.

- Enhanced Focus and Cognitive Clarity:
Coloring can also enhance focus and problem-solving skills. By engaging both sides of the brain, individuals experience improved mental clarity, a sense of calm, and a break from ruminative thoughts.

Case Study:
James, a high-stress professional, incorporated adult coloring into his evening routine as a way to unwind. Within weeks, he noticed a decrease in his evening anxiety. Reflecting on his experience, James said, "Coloring mandalas helped me quiet my mind and focus on something beautiful and calming. It became my favorite part of the day."

4. Ideas for Integrating Creative Outlets into a Holistic Healing Practice

Incorporating creative practices like tea rituals and coloring into daily routines can foster a balanced approach to managing stress and cultivating mental clarity. Here are a few ideas for making these activities part of a holistic healing practice:

- Daily Tea Meditation:
Set aside ten minutes each morning or evening for a mindful tea ritual. Use the time to focus solely on the preparation and sensory experience of the tea. Try to incorporate natural elements, like a bamboo whisk or a ceramic cup, to create a grounding environment.

- Mindful Coloring Routine:
Designate time each week for adult coloring, focusing on mandalas or intricate patterns. Choose colors intuitively, letting the process unfold without any particular goal. Reflect on the emotions that arise as you color to gain deeper insights into your emotional state.

- Combining Tea and Coloring for Deep Relaxation:
Pair a cup of tea with a coloring session for a soothing experience that engages multiple senses. The aroma and

warmth of the tea combined with the focused attention of coloring create a balanced ritual that promotes relaxation and calmness.

Case Study:

Sarah, an artist and mindfulness teacher, created a weekly group session combining tea rituals and adult coloring for her community. Participants reported a heightened sense of well-being and connection, appreciating the structured time for mindful creativity and relaxation. One participant, Maya, reflected, "The combination of tea and coloring felt like therapy. I left each session with a quiet mind and a sense of peace."

Key References and Resources

A variety of academic texts and expert insights support the benefits of tea and adult coloring for stress management:

- "The Book of Tea" by Kakuzo Okakura: Okakura's book explores the philosophy and artistry of tea, emphasizing the spiritual and calming aspects of tea ceremonies in Japan.
- "The Art of Mandala" by Suzy Andrick: This book provides insights into the practice of mandala coloring, detailing its benefits for mindfulness, focus, and emotional balance.
- "Flow: The Psychology of Optimal Experience" by Mihaly Csikszentmihalyi: Csikszentmihalyi's foundational work on flow states highlights how activities like adult coloring induce a mental state of focus and calm that contributes to overall well-being.
- Studies on L-theanine and Cortisol Reduction: Research has shown that L-theanine, a compound in tea,

significantly reduces cortisol levels, underscoring the physiological benefits of tea as a calming practice (Psychopharmacology, 2006).

Conclusion

The art of tea and adult coloring offer unique, meditative avenues for stress relief, encouraging mindfulness, calm, and self-expression. Through the intentional practice of tea preparation and mindful coloring, individuals can develop sustainable methods for managing stress and fostering clarity in their lives. As creative stress relief tools, these practices integrate seamlessly into a holistic healing approach, providing both emotional and physiological benefits that contribute to a sense of balance and inner peace.

Chapter 12: Practical Wisdom for Lifelong Holistic Wellness

As we seek to cultivate lasting well-being, adopting principles of practical wisdom can guide us toward a balanced and healthy life. This chapter explores the foundations of practical wisdom for managing stress and achieving overall health, provides insights into building a lifestyle centered on simplicity and inner peace, and offers a framework for creating a personalized, long-term holistic wellness plan.

1. Principles of Practical Wisdom for Stress Management and Overall Health

Practical wisdom, or phronesis in ancient philosophy, is the art of making sound, ethical, and mindful decisions in the face of life's challenges. Aristotle referred to practical wisdom as the key to a virtuous life, rooted in self-knowledge, mindfulness, and the ability to adapt to changing circumstances. In modern terms, practical wisdom entails a balanced approach to health, focusing on sustainable stress management and a commitment to holistic well-being.

Key Principles of Practical Wisdom in Wellness:

- Self-Awareness:
Knowing oneself is foundational to wise decision-making. Psychologist Carl Rogers emphasized the importance of self-awareness, stating, "The curious paradox is that when I accept myself just as I am, then I can change." By practicing self-reflection, individuals become attuned to their needs, making choices aligned with long-term well-being.

- Mindful Action:
Practical wisdom requires mindful action. Dr. Jon Kabat-Zinn, founder of Mindfulness-Based Stress Reduction (MBSR), explains that mindfulness allows us to "see things as they really are," enabling us to respond rather than react to stress.

- Adaptability and Resilience:
Resilience is essential for maintaining health. Research from Dr. Richard Davidson at the University of Wisconsin-Madison reveals that resilient individuals recover more quickly from stress and have better health outcomes.

By incorporating these principles, individuals can develop a practical, wise approach to managing stress and maintaining overall health.

Case Study:

Emma, a corporate manager facing burnout, found that practicing mindfulness and self-awareness helped her reframe her priorities. By setting boundaries and listening to her body's needs, she transformed her life and significantly reduced her stress levels. "The turning point for me was realizing that saying 'no' was an act of self-respect," Emma shared. "I had to start choosing actions that aligned with my values."

2. Building a Lifestyle Centered on Balance, Simplicity, and Inner Peace

Achieving holistic wellness requires a lifestyle that fosters balance, simplicity, and inner peace. Simplifying life—through reducing commitments, minimizing possessions, or cultivating peaceful spaces—can alleviate mental clutter and stress. The concept of minimalism and essentialism encourages a focus on what truly matters, leading to greater clarity and calmness.

Foundations of a Balanced, Simple Lifestyle:

- Simplicity in Daily Life:
Psychologist Barry Schwartz, author of The Paradox of Choice, argues that simplifying life reduces decision fatigue and enhances contentment. Simplifying routines and possessions minimizes distractions and cultivates a sense of peace.

- Connection with Nature:
Spending time in nature has proven benefits for mental health. A 2015 study published in Proceedings of the National Academy of Sciences found that walking in nature reduced rumination and improved mood, while Japanese practice of shinrin-yoku (forest bathing) has been shown to lower cortisol levels and boost immunity.

- Meaningful Relationships:
Prioritizing relationships that nurture us rather than drain us fosters a more balanced life. Dr. Brené Brown, a researcher on vulnerability and connection, notes, "Connection is why we're here; it is what gives purpose and meaning to our lives." Cultivating healthy boundaries and meaningful connections reduces stress and promotes inner peace.

Case Study:

Liam, a technology professional, felt overwhelmed by the constant influx of information in his life. Inspired by the simplicity movement, he reduced his digital consumption, limited his social media usage, and started spending time in nature. Over time, Liam noticed a significant reduction in anxiety and felt more grounded. "Less really is more," he reflected. "When I stripped away the unnecessary, I discovered a profound sense of peace."

3. Developing a Long-Term, Personalized Holistic Health Plan

A personalized health plan enables individuals to stay committed to wellness goals that support their unique needs. This plan encompasses physical, mental, and emotional health, encouraging a well-rounded approach to well-being. Creating a holistic plan involves identifying priorities, setting realistic goals, and incorporating practices that foster balance and resilience.

Steps to Create a Long-Term Holistic Health Plan:

- Identify Core Values and Wellness Goals:
Define what well-being means personally. Is it reducing stress, improving physical health, building emotional resilience, or a combination? Clarifying these values ensures that the wellness plan is relevant and sustainable.

- Choose Practices Aligned with Goals:
Practices may include regular exercise, mindfulness, nutrition, social activities, and self-care routines. Dr.

Dean Ornish, a pioneer in holistic health, advocates for an integrative approach to wellness, combining nutrition, exercise, stress management, and social support to promote heart health and overall well-being.

- Incorporate Routine Check-Ins:
Monitoring progress is essential for maintaining motivation. This can involve journaling, periodic health assessments, or discussing goals with a health professional. Routine check-ins allow for flexibility and adaptability, adjusting practices as life circumstances evolve.

Case Study:

Sarah, a teacher, struggled with chronic stress and insomnia. With the help of her therapist, she created a personalized wellness plan that included yoga, a balanced diet, and journaling. Six months later, Sarah noted significant improvements in her energy levels and mood. "I feel like I have my life back," she expressed, underscoring the power of a consistent and adaptable health plan.

4. Final Reflections on the Benefits of a Holistic Approach to Stress

Adopting a holistic approach to stress not only improves mental and physical health but also fosters a sense of purpose and fulfillment. Holistic wellness emphasizes treating the person as a whole, recognizing the interconnectedness of body, mind, and spirit. Rather than addressing symptoms in isolation, holistic wellness seeks to uncover root causes and cultivate resilience.

Long-Term Benefits of a Holistic Approach:

- Improved Mental and Emotional Resilience:
By practicing mindfulness, emotional regulation, and healthy coping mechanisms, individuals become better equipped to handle life's ups and downs. Holistic health practices foster emotional stability, reducing the risk of burnout and mental health issues.

- Enhanced Physical Health and Vitality:
Practices such as regular exercise, proper nutrition, and stress management contribute to physical wellness. Research has shown that holistic practices reduce inflammation, lower blood pressure, and strengthen the immune system.

- Sense of Purpose and Fulfillment:
Holistic wellness emphasizes self-discovery and connection to one's values. Through regular reflection and intentional living, individuals experience a deeper sense of purpose, which is essential for long-term happiness.

In her book Radical Acceptance, psychologist Tara Brach emphasizes the importance of self-compassion and acceptance in wellness. "Our deepest wounds surround our greatest gifts," she writes, illustrating that self-awareness and acceptance are essential elements in holistic wellness.

Key References and Resources

Several books and studies provide insights into practical wisdom, simplicity, and holistic health:

- "The Blue Zones" by Dan Buettner: This book explores the habits of the world's longest-lived communities, highlighting the importance of diet, movement, and social connections for holistic health.
- "Full Catastrophe Living" by Jon Kabat-Zinn: Kabat-Zinn's seminal work on mindfulness and stress reduction offers practical guidance on building a mindful and resilient lifestyle.
- "The Art of Happiness" by the Dalai Lama and Howard Cutler: This book explores how cultivating inner peace and balance contributes to long-term well-being, grounded in Buddhist philosophy and psychological insights.
- "Resilient" by Dr. Rick Hanson: Hanson's work on resilience provides actionable steps for building emotional strength, highlighting the benefits of practical wisdom and mindful practices in creating a balanced life.

Conclusion

Practical wisdom offers a pathway to lifelong holistic wellness by teaching us to make mindful, compassionate choices that support our well-being. Through simplicity, balance, and self-awareness, individuals can create a sustainable, fulfilling lifestyle. Embracing holistic wellness not only improves physical and mental health but also fosters a deep sense of peace, purpose, and resilience. By developing a personalized wellness plan and committing to mindful practices, we can approach life's challenges with confidence, ensuring that wellness remains a priority throughout all stages of life.

Chapter 13. Weekly plan with activities for stress reduction

This weekly plan combines physical activity, mindfulness, creative outlets, and reflection to help reduce stress. Each activity is designed to fit seamlessly into daily routines and build resilience and calm over time.

Table format

Day	Morning Activity	Midday Activity	Evening Activity
Monday	10-minute morning meditation or deep breathing exercises	Take a brisk 15-minute walk outside	Write in a gratitude journal, list three positive moments
Tuesday	Gentle yoga or stretching for 15 minutes	Practice mindful eating during lunch	20 minutes of adult coloring or creative activity
Wednesday	5 minutes of affirmations or positive visualization	Engage in a short walk and mindful breathing outdoors	Soothing herbal tea and a calming bath
Thursday	Morning journaling (set positive intentions for the day)	Short mindfulness meditation (5–10 minutes)	Read a chapter from a favorite book or

Day	Morning Activity	Midday Activity	Evening Activity
			inspiring text
Friday	Light physical exercise (walk, stretching, or dance)	Have a mindful check-in: assess the week's stressors	Listen to calming music and reflect on weekly progress
Saturday	Practice mindful tea or coffee ritual	Social activity or spend time in nature	Reflect on the week in a journal
Sunday	20-minute meditation or nature walk	Gentle stretching or restorative yoga	Plan upcoming week, set intentions for managing stress

Text format

Monday
- Morning: Begin with a 10-minute morning meditation or deep breathing exercises to set a calm tone for the day.
- Midday: Take a brisk 15-minute walk outside to refresh and reset your mind.
- Evening: Write in a gratitude journal, listing three positive moments from your day.

Tuesday

- Morning: Engage in gentle yoga or stretching for 15 minutes to relieve physical tension and promote relaxation.
- Midday: Practice mindful eating during lunch, focusing on the textures and flavors of each bite.
- Evening: Spend 20 minutes doing adult coloring or another creative activity to help unwind.

Wednesday
- Morning: Practice 5 minutes of affirmations or positive visualization to cultivate a positive mindset.
- Midday: Step outside for a short walk and practice mindful breathing to reduce midday stress.
- Evening: Enjoy a cup of soothing herbal tea and a calming bath for relaxation.

Thursday
- Morning: Journal briefly, setting positive intentions for the day ahead.
- Midday: Take a 5–10 minute mindfulness meditation break to refocus your mind.
- Evening: Read a chapter from a favorite book or inspiring text to ease into the night.

Friday
- Morning: Engage in light physical exercise, like walking, stretching, or dancing, to energize the body.
- Midday: Conduct a mindful check-in, reflecting on the week's stressors and achievements.
- Evening: Listen to calming music and reflect on the progress made throughout the week.

Saturday
- Morning: Practice a mindful tea or coffee ritual, savoring each sip to cultivate presence.

- Midday: Spend time in nature or engage in a social activity to feel refreshed and connected.
- Evening: Reflect on the week in a journal, noting any positive changes or areas for improvement.

Sunday
- Morning: Take a 20-minute nature walk or do a meditation session to promote inner peace.
- Midday: Engage in gentle stretching or restorative yoga to release tension.
- Evening: Plan the upcoming week, setting intentions to manage stress mindfully.

Chapter 14. Reference books for further research

These books cover a range of holistic approaches to stress reduction, from mindfulness and self-compassion to body-based healing, minimalism, and ancient wisdom. Each provides valuable insights for building a well-rounded stress management toolkit.

1. "The Body Keeps the Score" by Bessel van der Kolk
   Focuses on how trauma and stress affect the body and mind, offering insights into healing through somatic therapies and mindfulness.

2. "Full Catastrophe Living" by Jon Kabat-Zinn
   A comprehensive guide on Mindfulness-Based Stress Reduction (MBSR), with practices for managing stress and cultivating peace.

3. "Radical Acceptance" by Tara Brach
   Explores the power of self-compassion and acceptance as tools for reducing stress and finding inner calm.

4. "The Art of Happiness" by The Dalai Lama and Howard Cutler
   Combines Buddhist philosophy with modern psychology to offer insights into cultivating happiness and reducing stress.

5. "Eastern Body, Western Mind" by Anodea Judith
   Examines the chakra system as a framework for understanding and healing emotional stress and trauma.

6. "The Relaxation and Stress Reduction Workbook" by Martha Davis, Elizabeth Robbins Eshelman, and Matthew McKay
   A practical workbook with exercises and techniques for managing stress through relaxation, visualization, and mindfulness.

7. "The Power of Now" by Eckhart Tolle
   Focuses on the importance of staying present, discussing how mindfulness can alleviate stress and mental distress.

8. "The Healing Self" by Deepak Chopra and Rudolph Tanzi
   A guide to self-healing through lifestyle practices, emphasizing how stress reduction and self-care enhance physical health.

9. "When the Body Says No" by Gabor Maté
   Explores the mind-body connection and how unresolved stress can lead to illness, with guidance on healing holistically.

10. "The Untethered Soul" by Michael A. Singer
   Discusses how letting go of inner resistance and cultivating awareness can reduce stress and lead to personal freedom.

11. "The Mindful Way Workbook" by John Teasdale, Mark Williams, and Zindel Segal
   A workbook on using mindfulness-based cognitive therapy to alleviate stress, anxiety, and depression.

12. "Daring Greatly" by Brené Brown

Examines how embracing vulnerability and practicing self-compassion can relieve stress and build resilience.

13. "In Praise of Slowness" by Carl Honoré
   Analyzes the modern rush culture, encouraging readers to adopt a slower, more mindful approach to reduce stress.

14. "The Joy of Less" by Francine Jay
   Discusses minimalism as a path to reducing stress and finding clarity, focusing on simplicity in life.

15. "How to Relax" by Thich Nhat Hanh
   Offers meditative practices for achieving calm and balance, with accessible techniques for reducing stress.

16. "Resilient" by Rick Hanson
   Provides strategies to cultivate mental resilience and happiness, focusing on stress management through inner strengths.

17. "You Can Heal Your Life" by Louise Hay
   Explores the connection between thoughts and physical health, with affirmations for healing and stress relief.

18. "Chakra Healing" by Margarita Alcantara
   A guide on balancing chakras to enhance mental and emotional well-being, with exercises to reduce stress.

19. "Healing Yoga" by Loren Fishman and Ellen Saltonstall
   Covers yoga practices for stress relief and physical healing, focusing on alignment and breathing.

20. "The Four Agreements" by Don Miguel Ruiz
   Offers four principles to guide a stress-free and balanced life, rooted in Toltec wisdom and practical spirituality.

THE END